T0259261

Sleep and Psychiatry in Adults

Editors

JOHN H. HERMAN
MAX HIRSHKOWITZ

SLEEP MEDICINE CLINICS

www.sleep.theclinics.com

Consulting Editor
TEOFILO LEE-CHIONG Jr

March 2015 • Volume 10 • Number 1

ELSEVIER

1600 John F. Kennedy Boulevard • Suite 1800 • Philadelphia, Pennsylvania, 19103-2899

http://www.theclinics.com

SLEEP MEDICINE CLINICS Volume 10, Number 1
March 2015, ISSN 1556-407X, ISBN-13: 978-0-323-35666-4

Editor: Patrick Manley
Developmental Editor: Donald Mumford

© **2015 Elsevier Inc. All rights reserved.**

This periodical and the individual contributions contained in it are protected under copyright by Elsevier, and the following terms and conditions apply to their use:

Photocopying

Single photocopies of single articles may be made for personal use as allowed by national copyright laws. Permission of the Publisher and payment of a fee is required for all other photocopying, including multiple or systematic copying, copying for advertising or promotional purposes, resale, and all forms of document delivery. Special rates are available for educational institutions that wish to make photocopies for non-profit educational classroom use. For information on how to seek permission visit www.elsevier.com/permissions or call: (+44) 1865 843830 (UK)/(+1) 215 239 3804 (USA).

Derivative Works

Subscribers may reproduce tables of contents or prepare lists of articles including abstracts for internal circulation within their institutions. Permission of the Publisher is required for resale or distribution outside the institution. Permission of the Publisher is required for all other derivative works, including compilations and translations (please consult www.elsevier.com/permissions).

Electronic Storage or Usage

Permission of the Publisher is required to store or use electronically any material contained in this periodical, including any article or part of an article (please consult www.elsevier.com/permissions). Except as outlined above, no part of this publication may be reproduced, stored in a retrieval system or transmitted in any form or by any means, electronic, mechanical, photocopying, recording or otherwise, without prior written permission of the Publisher.

Notice

No responsibility is assumed by the Publisher for any injury and/or damage to persons or property as a matter of products liability, negligence or otherwise, or from any use or operation of any methods, products, instructions or ideas contained in the material herein. Because of rapid advances in the medical sciences, in particular, independent verification of diagnoses and drug dosages should be made. Although all advertising material is expected to conform to ethical (medical) standards, inclusion in this publication does not constitute a guarantee or endorsement of the quality or value of such product or of the claims made of it by its manufacturer.

Sleep Medicine Clinics (ISSN 1556-407X) is published quarterly by Elsevier Inc., 360 Park Avenue South, New York, NY 10010-1710. Months of issue are March, June, September and December. Business and Editorial Offices: 1600 John F. Kennedy Blvd., Ste. 1800, Philadelphia, PA 19103-2899. Customer Service Office: 3251 Riverport Lane, Maryland Heights, MO 63043. Periodicals postage paid at New York, NY and additional mailing offices. Subscription prices are $195.00 per year (US individuals), $95.00 (US residents), $406.00 (US institutions), $230.00 (Canadian individuals), $235.00 (international individuals), $135.00 (Canadian and international residents) and $452.00 (Canadian and international institutions). Foreign air speed delivery is included in all *Clinics* subscription prices. All prices are subject to change without notice. **POSTMASTER:** Send change of address to *Sleep Medicine Clinics*, Elsevier Health Sciences Division, Subscription Customer Service, 3251 Riverport Lane, Maryland Heights, MO 63043. Customer Service: **Tel: 1-800-654-2452 (U.S. and Canada); 314-447-8871 (outside U.S. and Canada). Fax: 314-447-8029. E-mail: journalscustomerservice-usa@elsevier.com (for print support); journalsonline support-usa@elsevier.com (for online support).**

Reprints. For copies of 100 or more of articles in this publication, please contact the Commercial Reprints Department, Elsevier Inc., 360 Park Avenue South, New York, NY 10010-1710. Tel.: 212-633-3874; Fax: 212-633-3820; E-mail: reprints@elsevier.com.

PROGRAM OBJECTIVE

The goal of *Sleep Clinics of North America* is to keep practicing physicians up to date with current clinical practice by providing timely articles reviewing the state of the art in patient care.

TARGET AUDIENCE

All practicing physicians and other healthcare professionals.

LEARNING OBJECTIVES

Upon completion of this activity, participants will be able to:

1. Discuss the use of non-benzodiazepine receptor agonists (BSRA) for insomnia.
2. Describe the relationship between stress, sleep deprivation and circadian disruption.
3. Recognize the role of anxiety and depression in sleep disturbances.

ACCREDITATION

The Elsevier Office of Continuing Medical Education (EOCME) is accredited by the Accreditation Council for Continuing Medical Education (ACCME) to provide continuing medical education for physicians.

The EOCME designates this enduring material for a maximum of 15 *AMA PRA Category 1 Credit(s)* ™. Physicians should claim only the credit commensurate with the extent of their participation in the activity.

All other health care professionals requesting continuing education credit for this enduring material will be issued a certificate of participation.

DISCLOSURE OF CONFLICTS OF INTEREST

The EOCME assesses conflict of interest with its instructors, faculty, planners, and other individuals who are in a position to control the content of CME activities. All relevant conflicts of interest that are identified are thoroughly vetted by EOCME for fair balance, scientific objectivity, and patient care recommendations. EOCME is committed to providing its learners with CME activities that promote improvements or quality in healthcare and not a specific proprietary business or a commercial interest.

The planning committee, staff, authors and editors listed below have identified no financial relationships or relationships to products or devices they or their spouse/life partner have with commercial interest related to the content of this CME activity:

Philip M. Becker, MD; Bei Bei, D Psych, PhD; Kathleen L. Benson, PhD, FAASM; Rebecca A. Bernert, PhD; Soledad Coo, PhD; Joseph M. Dzierzewski, PhD; Autumn M. Gallegos, PhD; Robert N. Glidewell, PsyD, CBSM; Allison G. Harvey, PhD; Patricia Haynes, PhD; Kristen Helm; John H. Herman, PhD; Max Hirshkowitz, PhD; Brynne Hunter; Katherine A. Kaplan, PhD; Ilia N. Karatsoreos, PhD; Daniel B. Kay, PhD; Sandy Lavery; Mahalakshmi Narayanan; Patrick Manley; Bruce S. McEwen, PhD; E. McPherson Botts, PsyD; Michael J. Murphy, MD, PhD; Michael R. Nadorff, PhD; William C. Orr, PhD; Wilfred R. Pigeon, PhD, CBSM; Adriane M. Soehner, PhD; Manya Somiah, MD; John Trinder, PhD.

The planning committee, staff, authors and editors listed below have identified financial relationships or relationships to products or devices they or their spouse/life partner have with commercial interest related to the content of this CME activity:

Teofilo Lee-Chiong Jr, MD has stock ownership, a research grant and an employment affiliation with Koninklijke Philips N.V. is a consultant/advisor for CareCore National and Elsevier; and has royalties/patents with Elsevier, Lippincott, Wiley, Oxford University and CreateSpace.

Michael J. Peterson, MD, PhD; is a consultant/advisor for MedicineNet, Inc. and Otsuka America Pharmaceutical, Inc.

UNAPPROVED/OFF-LABEL USE DISCLOSURE

The EOCME requires CME faculty to disclose to the participants:

1. When products or procedures being discussed are off-label, unlabelled, experimental, and/or investigational (not US Food and Drug Administration [FDA] approved) and
2. Any limitations on the information presented, such as data that are preliminary or that represent ongoing research, interim analyses, and/or unsupported opinions. Faculty may discuss information about pharmaceutical agents that is outside of FDA-approved labelling. This information is intended solely for CME and is not intended to promote off-label use of these medications. If you have any questions, contact the medical affairs department of the manufacturer for the most recent prescribing information.

TO ENROLL

To enroll in the Sleep Medicines Clinic Continuing Medical Education program, call customer service at 1-800-654-2452 or sign up online at http://www.theclinics.com/home/cme. The CME program is available to subscribers for an additional annual fee of USD $140.

METHOD OF PARTICIPATION

In order to claim credit, participants must complete the following:
1. Complete enrolment as indicated above.

2. Read the activity.
3. Complete the CME Test and Evaluation. Participants must achieve a score of 70% on the test. All CME Tests and Evaluations must be completed online.

CME INQUIRIES/SPECIAL NEEDS

For all CME inquiries or special needs, please contact elsevierCME@elsevier.com.

SLEEP MEDICINE CLINICS

ISSUES OF RELATED INTEREST

Clinics in Chest Medicine, Vol. 35, No.3 (September 2014)
Sleep-Disordered Breathing: Beyond Obstructive Sleep Apnea
Carolyn M. D'Ambrosio, MD, *Editor*

DOWNLOAD
Free App!

Review Articles
THE CLINICS

NOW AVAILABLE FOR YOUR iPhone and iPad

SLEEP MEDICINE CLINICS

FORTHCOMING ISSUES

June 2015
Sleep and Psychiatry in Children
John Herman and Max Hirshkowitz, Editors

September 2015
Restless Legs Syndrome and Movement Disorders
Denise Sharon, Editor

December 2015
Science of Circadian Rhythms
Phyllis Zee, Editor

RECENT ISSUES

December 2014
Evaluation of Sleep Complaints
Clete A. Kushida, Editor

September 2014
Sleep Hypoventilation: A State-of-the-Art Overview
Babak Mokhlesi, Editor

June 2014
Behavioral Aspects of Sleep Problems in Childhood and Adolescence
Judith A. Owens, Editor

ISSUES OF RELATED INTEREST

Clinics in Chest Medicine, Vol. 35, No.3 (September 2014)
Sleep-Disordered Breathing: Beyond Obstructive Sleep Apnea
Carolyn M. D'Ambrosio, MD, Editor

NOW AVAILABLE FOR YOUR iPhone and iPad

Contributors

CONSULTING EDITOR

TEOFILO LEE-CHIONG Jr, MD
Professor of Medicine, National Jewish
Health; Professor of Medicine, School of
Medicine, University of Colorado Denver,
Denver Colorado; Chief Medical Liaison,
Philips Respironics, Pennsylvania

EDITORS

JOHN H. HERMAN, PhD
Adjunct Professor, University of Texas
Southwestern Medical Center at Dallas,
Dallas, Texas

MAX HIRSHKOWITZ, PhD
Professor Emeritus, Baylor College of
Medicine, Houston, Texas; Consulting
Professor, Stanford University School of
Medicine, Palo Alto, California

AUTHORS

PHILIP M. BECKER, MD
Clinical Professor, Department of Psychiatry,
University of Texas Southwestern Medical
Center at Dallas; President, Sleep Medicine
Associates of Texas, Dallas, Texas

BEI BEI, DPsych, PhD
Melbourne School of Psychological Sciences,
University of Melbourne, Parkville, Victoria;
School of Psychological Sciences, Monash
University, Australia

KATHLEEN L. BENSON, PhD, FAASM
Research Associate, Neuroimaging Section,
McLean Hospital, Belmont; Department of
Psychiatry, Harvard Medical School, Boston,
Massachusetts

REBECCA A. BERNERT, PhD
Department of Psychiatry and Behavioral
Sciences, Stanford University School of
Medicine, Stanford, California

SOLEDAD COO, PhD
Melbourne School of Psychological Sciences,
University of Melbourne, Parkville, Victoria,
Australia

JOSEPH M. DZIERZEWSKI, PhD
Assistant Professor, David Geffen School of
Medicine, University of California, Los Angeles;
Geriatric Research, Education, and Clinical
Center, VA Greater Los Angeles Healthcare
System, Los Angeles, California

AUTUMN M. GALLEGOS, PhD
Department of Veterans Affairs VISN 2
Center of Excellence for Suicide
Prevention, Canandaigua VA Medical Center,
Canandaigua; Sleep and Neurophysiology
Research Laboratory, Department of
Psychiatry, University of Rochester Medical
Center, Rochester, New York

ROBERT N. GLIDEWELL, PsyD, CBSM
President and CEO, Behavioral Sleep
Medicine, LLC, Colorado Springs; Affiliate
Faculty, National Jewish Health, Denver,
Colorado

ALLISON G. HARVEY, PhD
Department of Psychology,
University of California Berkeley,
Berkeley, California

PATRICIA HAYNES, PhD
Assistant Professor, Department of Psychiatry, University of Arizona, Tucson, Arizona

KATHERINE A. KAPLAN, PhD
Department of Psychiatry, Stanford University School of Medicine, Psychiatry and Behavioral Sciences, Stanford, California

ILIA N. KARATSOREOS, PhD
Department of Integrative Physiology and Neuroscience, Washington State University, Pullman, Washington

DANIEL B. KAY, PhD
Postdoctoral Scholar, Department of Psychiatry, University of Pittsburgh, Pittsburgh

BRUCE S. MCEWEN, PhD
The Alfred E. Mirsky Professor, Head, Harold and Margaret Milliken Hatch Laboratory of Neuroendocrinology, The Rockefeller University, New York, New York

E. MCPHERSON BOTTS, PsyD
Psychologist, Private Practice, Colorado Springs, Colorado

MICHAEL J. MURPHY, MD, PhD
Department of Psychiatry, Massachusetts General Hospital, Boston; McLean Hospital, Belmont, Massachusetts

MICHAEL R. NADORFF, PhD
Department of Psychology, Mississippi State University, Starkville, Mississippi

WILLIAM C. ORR, PhD
Clinical Professor of Medicine, University of Oklahoma Health Sciences Center; President Emeritus, Lynn Health Science Institute, Oklahoma City, Oklahoma

MICHAEL J. PETERSON, MD, PhD
Assistant Professor; Director of Hospital Psychiatric Services, Department of Psychiatry, University of Wisconsin School of Medicine and Public Health, Madison, Wisconsin

WILFRED R. PIGEON, PhD, CBSM
Department of Veterans Affairs VISN 2 Center of Excellence for Suicide Prevention, Canandaigua VA Medical Center, Canandaigua; Sleep and Neurophysiology Research Laboratory, Department of Psychiatry, University of Rochester Medical Center, Rochester; Department of Veterans Affairs Center for Integrated Healthcare, Syracuse VA Medical Center, Syracuse, New York

ADRIANE M. SOEHNER, PhD
Department of Psychiatry, University of Pittsburgh School of Medicine, Western Psychiatric Institute and Clinic, Pittsburgh, Pennsylvania

MANYA SOMIAH, MD
Research Associate, Sleep Medicine Associates of Texas, Dallas, Texas

JOHN TRINDER, PhD
Melbourne School of Psychological Sciences, University of Melbourne, Parkville, Victoria, Australia

Contents

Sleep Deprivation and Circadian Disruption: Stress, Allostasis, and Allostatic Load 1

Bruce S. McEwen and Ilia N. Karatsoreos

> Sleep has important homeostatic functions, and circadian rhythms organize physiology and behavior on a daily basis to insure optimal function. Sleep deprivation and circadian disruption can be stressors, enhancers of other stressors that have consequences for the brain and many body systems. Whether the origins of circadian disruption and sleep disruption and deprivation are from anxiety, depression, shift work, long-distance air travel, or a hectic lifestyle, there are consequences that impair brain functions and contribute to the cumulative wear and tear on body systems caused by too much stress and/or inefficient management of the systems that promote adaptation.

Sleep in the Context of Healthy Aging and Psychiatric Syndromes 11

Daniel B. Kay and Joseph M. Dzierzewski

> Humans spend approximately one-third of their lives asleep. Whether due to evolutionary or ontogenetic factors, sleep and psychiatric disorders change with age. Although much of sleep remains an enigma, sleep research is experiencing an exponential increase in its understanding of the causes, correlates, and consequences of sleep disturbances. Although the relationship between age-related sleep and psychiatric conditions is a common clinical observation, empirical investigations remain scarce. Thus, treating patients with symptoms of sleep disorders in the context of psychiatric conditions remains a challenge. This article reviews the state-of-the-science of sleep disorders in the context of psychiatric conditions in late-life.

Sleep Disturbances in Depression 17

Michael J. Murphy and Michael J. Peterson

> Major depressive disorder is frequently accompanied by sleep disturbances such as insomnia or hypersomnia and polysomnographic sleep findings of increased rapid-eye-movement sleep and decreased slow wave sleep. For many patients, insomnia persists even after mood symptoms have been adequately treated. These patients have poorer outcomes than patients without sleep problems. These outcomes suggest that overlapping neural mechanisms regulate sleep and mood. Treatment of these patients can incorporate sedating antidepressants, nonbenzodiazepine γ-aminobutyric acid agonists, and cognitive behavioral therapy. Sleep restriction has been found to improve mood in depressed patients; however, the benefits typically disappear after recovery sleep.

Sleep and Mood During Pregnancy and the Postpartum Period 25

Bei Bei, Soledad Coo, and John Trinder

> During the perinatal period, compromises in sleep duration and quality are commonly reported by women and confirmed by objective measurements of sleep.

Self-reported poor sleep has been associated with concurrent mood disturbance and with increased risk for future mood problems during pregnancy and the postpartum period. Findings on the relationship between objectively measured sleep and mood in perinatal women have been mixed. This article reviews the literature on the nature of and contributing factors to perinatal sleep disturbance, the relationship between sleep and mood, and intervention studies that aim to improve maternal sleep.

Sleep Disturbances and Suicide Risk

Rebecca A. Bernert and Michael R. Nadorff

Suicide occurs in the presence of psychiatric illness, and is associated with biological, psychological, and social risk factors. Insomnia symptoms and nightmares appear to present elevated risk for suicidal ideation, attempts, and death by suicide. Failure to account for the presence of psychopathology and frequent use of single item assessments of sleep and suicidal ideation are common methodological problems in this literature. Preliminary research, addressing these issues, suggests that subjective sleep complaints may confer independent risk for suicidal behaviors.

Posttraumatic Stress Disorder and Sleep

Wilfred R. Pigeon and Autumn M. Gallegos

The purpose of this article is to provide a brief overview of sleep in the context of posttraumatic stress disorder (PTSD) and focus on the treatment of the most common sleep disorders encountered by patients with PTSD: insomnia and nightmares. The effects of the standard treatments for PTSD are discussed along with a review of available treatments for insomnia and nightmares. Particular emphasis is placed on nonpharmacologic treatments for these sleep disorders and how they may be adapted for delivery to patients with PTSD.

Sleep in Schizophrenia: Pathology and Treatment

Kathleen L. Benson

Both subjective and objective assessments of sleep patterns in schizophrenia include a wide range of dyssomnias, with insomnia being the most frequently cited. Early and middle insomnia can range from mild disruption to total sleeplessness. Severe insomnia is a prodromal sign of clinical exacerbation or relapse. In general, most antipsychotic agents (APs) ameliorate this insomnia. However, in some schizophrenics APs can be associated with residual insomnia or with significant daytime somnolence. Furthermore, in some schizophrenics APs can induce or exacerbate comorbid sleep disorders such as restless legs syndrome, sleep-disordered breathing, and parasomnias such as sleepwalking.

Non–Benzodiazepine Receptor Agonists for Insomnia

Philip M. Becker and Manya Somiah

Because of proven efficacy, reduced side effects, and less concern about addiction, non–benzodiazepine receptor agonists (non-BzRA) have become the most commonly prescribed hypnotic agents to treat onset and maintenance insomnia. First-line treatment is cognitive-behavioral therapy. When pharmacologic treatment is indicated, non-BzRA are first-line agents for the short-term and long-term management of transient and chronic insomnia related to adjustment, psychophysiologic, primary, and secondary causation. In this article, the benefits and risks of non-BzRA are reviewed, and the selection of a hypnotic agent is defined, based on efficacy, pharmacologic profile, and adverse events.

This article provides an overview of cognitive behavioral therapy (CBT) for insomnia and depression. Included is a discussion of how CBT for insomnia affects depression symptoms and how CBT for depression affects insomnia symptoms. The extant literature is reviewed on ways that depression/insomnia comorbidity moderates CBT response. The article concludes with an introduction to cognitive behavioral social rhythm therapy, a group therapy that integrates tenets of CBT for both disorders.

Hypnosis has been used to manage insomnia and disorders of arousal. The alteration in the state of consciousness produced during hypnotic trance is more similar to relaxed reverie than sleep. Hypnosis typically occurs in a state of repose and the accomplished subject may have no recollection of the experience during a trance, 2 commonalities with sleep. Because hypnosis allows for relaxation, increased suggestibility, posthypnotic suggestion, imagery rehearsal, access to preconscious cognitions and emotions, and cognitive restructuring, disorders of sleep such as the insomnias, parasomnias, and related mood or anxiety disorders can be amenable to this therapeutic intervention.

Concurrent clinical presentation of insomnia and anxiety is frequent in clinical practice. The onset and course of anxiety and insomnia are intimately related; traditional conceptualizations of insomnia as secondary to anxiety are no longer clinically viable. Evolving evidence suggests a relationship between these two conditions that is complex and reciprocal and that evolves over time. In terms of diagnosis and management, unless initial assessment and intervention are initiated in the earliest stages of illness, emerging opinion supports recognition of co-occurring anxiety and insomnia as independent comorbid conditions with each condition likely requiring targeted therapeutic attention to achieve optimal therapeutic outcomes.

Bipolar disorder is a severe and chronic disorder, ranked in the top 10 leading causes of disability worldwide. Sleep disturbances are strongly coupled with inter-episode dysfunction and symptom worsening in bipolar disorder. Experimental studies suggest that sleep deprivation can trigger manic relapse. There is evidence that sleep deprivation can have an adverse impact on emotion regulation the following day. The clinical management of the sleep disturbances experienced by bipolar patients, including insomnia, hypersomnia delayed sleep phase, and irregular sleep-wake schedule, may include medication approaches, psychological interventions, light therapies and sleep deprivation.

Preface
Sleep and Psychiatry in Adults

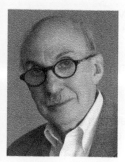
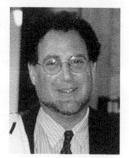

John H. Herman, PhD   Max Hirshkowitz, PhD
Editors

Sleep and psychiatric disorders often appear inextricably linked. Psychiatric symptoms exacerbation commonly precedes, accompanies, or follows mild to severely disrupted sleep. This connection occurs across the full spectrum of psychiatric disorders and in all age groups. This intriguing relationship raises several questions:

- Is worsening of sleep the progenitor or result of an exacerbation of psychiatric decompensation?
- Do sleep disruption and psychiatric disorders share common brain structures or neurochemical processes?
- Is the above cause and effect or comorbidity?

To explore these issues, we began by examining sleep disturbance, circadian disturbance, and stress. Regardless of what we think stress actually entails, sleep deprivation represents a major stressor that increases allosteric load. Furthermore, virtually every biological system depends on the sleep homeostatic process for normal function.

This issue leads off with an insightful article describing increased allosteric load with sleep deprivation disrupting normal brain and bodily function. Next, Drs Kay and Dzierzewski examine sleep throughout the lifespan in the context of normal aging as compared with the development of psychiatric syndromes. Sleep quality deteriorates far more significantly in the presence of a psychiatric comorbidity. In the third article, authors examine the relationship between sleep and affective disorders, with focus on the critical role of restoring normal sleep as part of the process for treating depression. Exploring this

relationship further, Bei and colleagues examine self-reported poor sleep and depressed mood during the perinatal period. Importantly, perceived poor sleep is a risk factor for both antepartum and postpartum mood disturbances.

Suicidality represents a major concern in patients with depression. Bernert reviews the evidence linking insomnia and/or increased frequency of nightmares with suicidal ideation, suicide attempts, and successful suicide completion in both anxiety and mood disorders. Insomnia and nightmares both frequently accompany PTSD and Dr Pigeon-Gallegos nicely describes that association. Treatment options, including CBT for insomnia, image rehearsal therapy, and prasozin for nightmares, are also described. Dr Benson shows us how schizophrenia is frequently comorbid with severe insomnia. Furthermore, she discusses how an episode of sleeplessness can represent a prodromal indication of an emerging decompensation episode or relapse.

The remainder of this issue addresses sleep-disturbance treatments and management, both pharmacologic and behavioral. Dr Becker and colleagues review the indications and recommendations for nonbenzodiazepine receptor agonists. Dr Haynes describes cognitive behavioral therapy of insomnia and Dr Becker reviews the use of hypnosis in insomnia associated with a mental disorder. Because treatment information will potentially provide practical clinical approaches, we present not just straightforward interventions but also ones that involve complex interactions that are notoriously difficult to manage (see article by Drs Glidewell, Botts, and Orr). Finally,

Sleep Med Clin 10 (2015) xiii–xiv
http://dx.doi.org/10.1016/j.jsmc.2014.12.001
1556-407X/15/$ – see front matter © 2015 Published by Elsevier Inc.

treatment approach for patients with relevant co-morbid illnesses (for example, bipolar disorder) is exemplified in the article by Dr Harvey and colleagues.

It is our hope that this issue will prove helpful to practitioners involved in treating psychiatric disorders with comorbid sleep disturbances. Understanding the relationship between sleep disorders and psychiatric problems represents an initial step. Discussing therapeutic approaches, especially in complex cases, sometimes provides the insight needed to make clinical progress. Ultimately our goal is to improve care for our patients struggling with these overlapping disorders.

John H. Herman, PhD
University of Texas Southwestern
Medical Center at Dallas
Dallas, TX, USA

Max Hirshkowitz, PhD
Baylor College of Medicine
Houston, TX, USA

Stanford University School of Medicine
Palo Alto, CA, USA

E-mail addresses:
john.herman.phd@gmail.com (J.H. Herman)
max.hirshkowitz@gmail.com (M. Hirshkowitz)

Sleep Deprivation and Circadian Disruption
Stress, Allostasis, and Allostatic Load

Bruce S. McEwen, PhD[a],*, Ilia N. Karatsoreos, PhD[b]

KEYWORDS

- Sleep deprivation • Hippocampus • Allostasis • Allostatic load • Glycogen • Oxidative stress
- Pro-inflammatory cytokines • Circadian disruption

KEY POINTS

- Allostatic load/overload refers to the cumulative wear and tear on body systems caused by too much stress and/or inefficient management of the systems that promote adaptation through allostasis.
- Circadian disruption is a broad problem that alters allostasis and elevates allostatic load, affecting brain and body systems. Sleep deprivation is an all-too-common example of a process that includes circadian disruption.
- Even a few days of sleep deprivation or circadian misalignment in young healthy volunteers have been reported to increase appetite and caloric intake, increase levels of pro-inflammatory cytokines, decrease parasympathetic and increase sympathetic tone, increase blood pressure, increase evening cortisol levels, as well as elevate insulin and blood glucose.
- Chronic circadian disruption and reduced sleep time are associated with elevated cortisol, increased obesity, and reduced volume of the temporal lobe.
- Mood disorders involve disrupted circadian rhythmicity and altered sleep-wake patterns; yet, acute sleep deprivation can have rapid antidepressant effects and manipulating the timing of the secretion or exogenous administration of melatonin can be beneficial in mood disorders.
- Repeated stress in animal models causes brain regions involved in memory and emotions, such as hippocampus, amygdala, and prefrontal cortex, to undergo structural remodeling with the result that memory is impaired and anxiety and aggression are increased. Structural and functional MRI studies in depression and Cushing disease, as well as anxiety disorders and in air crews with jet lag, provide evidence that the human brain may be similarly affected.
- Brain regions such as the hippocampus are sensitive to glucose and insulin, and both type I and type II diabetes are associated with cognitive impairment and (for type II diabetes) an increased risk for Alzheimer disease. Insofar as poor sleep and circadian disruption also exacerbate metabolic dysregulation as well as contribute to other aspects of physiologic dysregulation, they must be considered contributors to risk for dementia.
- Animal models of chronic sleep deprivation indicate that memory is impaired along with depletion of glycogen stores and increases in oxidative stress and free-radical production.

[a] Harold and Margaret Milliken Hatch Laboratory of Neuroendocrinology, The Rockefeller University, 1230 York Avenue, New York, NY 10065, USA; [b] Department of Integrative Physiology and Neuroscience, Washington State University, 1815 Ferdinand's Lane, Pullman, WA 99164-6520, USA
* Corresponding author.
E-mail address: mcewen@mail.rockefeller.edu

Sleep Med Clin 10 (2015) 1–10
http://dx.doi.org/10.1016/j.jsmc.2014.11.007
1556-407X/15/$ – see front matter © 2015 Elsevier Inc. All rights reserved.

INTRODUCTION

Anecdotally, there can be little doubt that sleep plays a role in maintaining a good mood and cognitive acuity. Sleep deprivation one night followed by "getting a good night's sleep" on the next clearly impacts neurobehavioral function as well as promotes physiologic balance and resilience. These subjective impressions are supported by numerous laboratory studies of endocrine function and metabolism as well as from investigations of sleep deprivation effects on cognitive and neural function, including research on the brain that shows a variety of substantial changes resulting from sleep restriction, with reversal after recovery sleep. Similarly, being "out of phase" with local time, be it from a week of nightshift work following a week of dayshift work, or transmeridian air travel across multiple time zones, demonstrates that there are both neural and physiologic effects of internal circadian (daily) time being misaligned with external environmental time. This article reviews selected aspects of the current state of knowledge in these areas and then evaluates what is known using the model of allostasis and allostatic load that emphasizes the "wear and tear" on the brain and body from coping with stress.

ALLOSTASIS AND ALLOSTATIC OVERLOAD

The maintenance of homeostasis, defined as those aspects of physiology that must remain stable to keep us alive (eg, oxygen tension, body temperature, pH), is an active process requiring coordinated action of many different systems, including the autonomic nervous system and neuroendocrine and immune systems. This active process is called "allostasis" or "maintaining stability through change."[1–3] Allostatic mediators work as a nonlinear, sometimes reciprocating, network (**Fig. 1**), meaning that too much or too little of each mediator can perturb the entire network, leading to harmful consequences. Take for example the relationship between cytokines and the glucocorticoids. Pro-inflammatory cytokines stimulate the production of cortisol, which then suppresses inflammatory cytokine production.[4,5] Similarly, increased activity of the sympathetic nervous system increases pro-inflammatory cytokine production, whereas parasympathetic activity has the opposite effect.[6,7] This balance is particularly important, as during an infection, the pro-inflammatory response that is essential to mounting an immune defense is normally contained by cortisol and also by parasympathetic activity.[4,6] Inadequate containment can lead to septic shock and death. Treatment with cortisol, or elevation of parasympathetic activity, is a pathway that can reduce the exaggerated inflammatory response.[4] However, at the opposite extreme, too much cortisol can suppress pro-inflammatory responses, thus compromising immune defenses.[4,8]

Allostatic overload, which is wear and tear produced by imbalances in the mediators of allostasis, is perfectly illustrated by these 2 examples: too much or too little activity of certain mediators of allostasis.[9] Other examples of allostatic overload include conditions such as hypertension, atherosclerosis, diabetes, and the metabolic syndrome as well as stress-induced remodeling in brain regions that support memory, executive function, and anxiety.[3,10] One of the key mediators

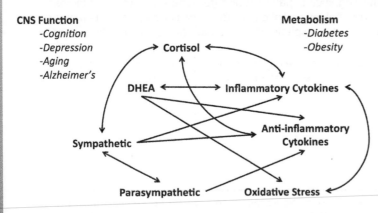

CNS Function
-Cognition
-Depression
-Aging
-Alzheimer's

Metabolism
-Diabetes
-Obesity

Cardiovascular Function
-Endothelial cell damage
-Atherosclerosis

Immune Function
-Enhancement
-Suppression

Fig. 1. Nonlinear network of mediators of allostasis involved in the stress response. Arrows indicate that each system regulates the others in a reciprocal manner, creating a nonlinear network. Moreover, there are multiple pathways for regulation (eg, inflammatory cytokine production is negatively regulated via anti-inflammatory cytokines as well as via parasympathetic and glucocorticoid pathways), whereas sympathetic activity increases inflammatory cytokine production. Parasympathetic activity, in turn, contains sympathetic activity. CNS, central nervous system; DHEA, dehydroepiandrosterone. (Adapted from Karatsoreos IN, McEwen BS. Psychobiological allostasis: resistance, resilience and vulnerability. Trends Cogn Sci 2011;15:576–84; with permission.)

of allostasis is cortisol (corticosterone in rodent species), and conditions in which corticosteroid balance is affected lead to many such changes in physiologic function and brain structure. Cushing disease and anxiety/depressive disorders are 2 such conditions that affect multiple allostatic mediators, including the corticosteroids.

Cushing disease, broadly defined as hypercortisolemia induced by organic (eg, pituitary or adrenal tumor) or iatrogenic (eg, high doses of corticosteroids to reduce inflammation) factors, is accompanied by several cognitive and emotional symptoms, including depression. Intriguingly, depressive symptoms can be relieved by surgical correction of hypercortisolemia (see[11]). In major depressive illness as well as in Cushing disease, the duration of the illness and not the age of the subject predicts a progressive reduction in hippocampal volume and is observed by structural MRI.[12] Moreover, there are a variety of other anxiety-related disorders, such as posttraumatic stress disorder (PTSD), in which atrophy of the hippocampus has been reported,[13,14] suggesting that this is a common process reflecting chronic imbalance in the activity of adaptive systems. These chronic imbalances include the hypothalamic-pituitary-adrenal (HPA) axis, and also endogenous neurotransmitters, such as glutamate.[12] Metabolic symptoms are also reported in both Cushing and major depression, as both are associated with chronic elevation of cortisol that results in gradual loss of minerals from bone, and increases in abdominal obesity.

CIRCADIAN DISRUPTION AND ALLOSTATIC LOAD AND OVERLOAD

When exploring how the brain and body are affected by stress, it is often overlooked that they may be directly regulated by time of day. All of the systems that are modulators of allostasis show rhythms of activity over the sleep-wake cycle. For instance, Cortisol (corticosterone in rodents; CORT) shows a clear circadian pattern, with the peak of CORT occurring just before waking in both nocturnal animals (such as rats and mice) and diurnal animals (such as humans). Circadian rhythms are observed in almost all physiologic measures, including endocrine and immune mediators.[15–17] Many of these factors are also impacted by sleep deprivation, as is discussed later. The circadian system in mammals is centered in the suprachiasmatic nucleus (SCN), with both neural and hormonal projections throughout the brain and body, and impacting many of the systems involved in mediating allostasis; disruption of the circadian system can place the organism into a state of high allostatic load. Indeed, if circadian patterns of CORT are disrupted by adrenalectomy (ADX) and tonic replacement of CORT via a pellet implant providing no diurnal rhythm, this results in a "sluggish" HPA axis response, with poor shutoff of adrenocorticotropic hormone following termination of a stressor, in contrast to the situation in which the ADX animal drinks CORT in the water in a diurnal pattern.[18] That CORT is also able to reset peripheral oscillators in other body tissues lends credence to an important relationship between disrupted rhythms and allostatic load; this is important because circadian disruption (CD; eg, shift work and jet lag) and sleep deprivation are not uncommon in the modern world and constitute an increasing health concern.[19,20]

The master circadian clock is located in the SCN of the hypothalamus and drives all rhythms in physiology and behavior.[21–23] In addition to the master SCN clock, "peripheral" circadian clocks, in tissues throughout the body, serve to set local time. These peripheral clocks are synchronized to the SCN by a multitude of signals, including glucocorticoids, which are able to "reset" some peripheral clocks in the brain and body (eg, liver), but not others.[24] In the brain, it has been shown that rhythms in glucocorticoids modulate clock protein expression in the oval nucleus of the bed nucleus of the stria terminalis as well as the central amygdala (CEA).[25] It is also known that the basolateral nuclei of the amygdala and the dentate gyrus of the hippocampus express opposite diurnal rhythms of PERIOD2 (a core clock component) when compared with the CEA, and that the CEA rhythm is further influenced by ADX.[26] The differential regulation of cellular rhythms in different brain regions is of particular interest when considering "healthy" regulation of HPA function requires rhythmic glucocorticoids, as discussed above.[18] It is posited that if efficient regulation of the HPA axis is a hallmark of a "healthy" response, then disrupted circadian patterns (or, in this case, a lack of a pattern) can result in an unhealthy regulation of the HPA and thus could contribute to allostatic load.[27] Thus, both disruption of the HPA axis and disruption of circadian rhythms could have interacting effects and contribute to shifts in resilience and vulnerability.

Both descriptive and epidemiologic studies show that individuals who suffer from repeated chronic circadian misalignment show negative physiologic, neural, and behavioral effects. In humans, a study of flight crews showed that those who endure more bouts of jet lag (transmeridian, short recovery crews) show shrunken medial temporal lobes, increased reaction time, and poorer performance in visual-spatial cognitive tasks compared with long recovery crews. In addition to the neurobehavioral effects, short-recovery individuals displayed a significant correlation between salivary cortisol levels and medial temporal cortex volume, whereas this effect was not observed in long recovery crews. Thus, rapid and repeated shifting of the circadian clock through jet lag is related to reductions in volume of the medial temporal lobe and shifts in behavioral performance on attentional tasks. Moreover, the brain effects are correlated with plasma cortisol levels. What is the significance of these neural and physiologic changes? It is intriguing to speculate that perhaps such shrunken temporal lobes may impart decreased resilience to negative outcomes of stress, as has been observed in PTSD.[28,29] In addition, sleep deprivation seems to increase the amygdalar response to negative emotional stimuli because of an amygdala-prefrontal disconnect.[30] Such effects could also exacerbate cardiovascular reactivity, which may contribute to pathophysiology.[31–33] Sleep deprivation studies have investigated the effects of chronic deprivation on cognitive performance, in both animal and human subjects, but in many cases, the stressful effects of the methods used to induce sleep deprivation confound these studies. Thus, a different approach must be applied to help disentangle these effects.

To directly probe how disruption of the circadian clock affects neurobehavioral function, new models need to be applied, and new hypotheses need to be tested. Karatsoreos and coworkers[34] characterized a mouse model of chronic CD that has provided several novel insights. This model induces disruption by housing mice in a light-dark cycle of 20 hours (10 hours light, 10 hours dark) compared with laboratory standard 24-hour cycles. After only 5 weeks of this environmental disruption, CD mice begin showing metabolic signs of allostatic load, including increased weight, adiposity, and leptin levels. A significant effect is also observed in glucose metabolism, because CD mice also show an imbalance between insulin and plasma glucose, suggesting development of a prediabetic state. Strikingly, the observed metabolic changes are accompanied by changes in prefrontal cortex cellular morphology, mirroring those observed in chronic stress. CD animals show shrunken and less complex apical dendritic trees of cells in layer II/III of the medial prefrontal cortex,[34] with no apparent effects on basal dendrites. CD animals further show behavioral abnormalities, with marked cognitive rigidity in a modified Morris water maze. Specifically, CD mice demonstrate normal performance on the learning phase of the initial task, but are slower to adapt to the hidden platform being moved to a novel location. These changes were mostly due to the mice making more perseverative errors by returning to the original location of the platform.[34] In addition to the cognitive flexibility problems, CD mice display what may be considered an "impulsive"-like phenotype in the light-dark box, while not showing any overt anxiety-like phenotype.[34] Taken in a wider context, these effects of CD are remarkably similar to those observed in 21 days of chronic restraint stress in rodents, which results in morphologic simplification of prefrontal cortical neurons and impairment in prefrontal mediated behaviors, such as attentional set-shifting or other working memory tasks.[35–37] When discussing such models of CD, it is important to note that, just as total hippocampal lesions provided insight into the role of this brain structure in learning and memory, circadian models are purposefully "exotic" (ie, shortened 20-hour days are not expected to become a common occurrence in human society). These models should provide important proof-of-principle concepts that should set the stage for more ecologically relevant and more refined models to be developed.

The specific mechanisms by which disrupted circadian clocks cause changes in brain, behavior, and peripheral physiology remain unknown. One hypothesis is that disrupted light-dark cycles lead to a gradual loss of cohesion between circadian clocks in the brain (eg, the SCN) and those in the body (eg, liver). This loss of cohesion results in central and peripheral oscillators eventually becoming out of phase with each other, creating internal desynchrony. In the brain, this could lead to changes in synchrony between various nodes of a neural circuit (eg, the prefrontal cortex and amygdala drifting out of phase). Over many cycles, such loss of cohesion could lead to changes in neurobehavioral function (as evidenced in[34]). In addition to long-term, chronic CD, shorter durations of CD could lead to changes in these circuits that make them more vulnerable to further insult and could be a more insidious mechanism of circuit level disruption, setting the stage for other stressors (eg, metabolic stress, immune stress) to overwhelm an already compromised network. Extending this model to the periphery, disruption of peripheral body clocks could lead to changes in the way the stress system responds to environmental or psychological stressors. Together, this model illustrates how CD could lead to neural circuits becoming more vulnerable to insult as well as pathways by which disruption could compromise allostatic responses engaged to help an organism adapt to environmental challenge. In this schema, CD effects may be similar to the diathesis-stress models, which could explain many of the epidemiologic findings of increased risk for development of psychiatric, cardiovascular, or other physiologic syndromes in populations undergoing chronic CD, such as shift workers.[20,38–40]

METABOLIC AND HORMONAL RESPONSES TO SLEEP DEPRIVATION AND CIRCADIAN DISRUPTION

Sleep deprivation produces an allostatic overload that can have deleterious consequences. Increases in blood pressure, decreases in parasympathetic tone, and increases in evening cortisol are all observed after only 4 hours of sleep deprivation. Metabolic effects of this short-duration deprivation also include increased insulin levels and increased appetite, possibly through the elevation of ghrelin, a pro-appetitive hormone, and decreased levels of leptin.[41–43] These short-term effects of sleep deprivation are significant when one considers epidemiologic evidence showing that reduced sleep duration is associated with increased body mass and obesity in the NHANES study.[44] However, these relationships are by no means simple. For instance, in adolescents, sleep reduction is associated with measurable changes in insulin sensitivity,[45] whereas durations of sleep longer than average are not associated with such changes. Similarly, a study by St-Onge and colleagues[46] in adults suggests that short-term sleep deprivation is not the cause of altered insulin sensitivity per se, but instead may contribute to overeating, potentially via different mechanisms in men and women. An important study by Vetrivelan and colleagues[47] showed that chronic partial sleep loss in a rat model of spontaneous short sleep did not lead to changes in metabolism, with the authors suggesting that observed effects on metabolism in sleep deprivation studies may instead be due to other factors, such as CD, changes in diet, or reduced activity levels. This work is clearly supported by the earlier CD work of Karatsoreos and McEwen,[27] in which mice that were circadian-disrupted, but not explicitly sleep-deprived, gained weight and had altered levels of plasma insulin and leptin.

Sleep deprivation also has marked effects on other circulating messengers, in addition to metabolic effects. Specifically, immune mediators are also altered following sleep deprivation. Pro-inflammatory cytokine levels are increased, along with deterioration in performance as measured by tests of psychomotor vigilance, and this has been reported to result from a modest sleep restriction to 6 hours per night.[48] In humans, poor sleep and sleep deprivation in aging women have been associated with elevated levels of interleukin (IL)-6.[49] Thus, clear links exist between sleep deprivation, CD, and neurobehavioral, metabolic, and immune function.

SLEEP DEPRIVATION AND CIRCADIAN DISRUPTION IN MOOD DISORDERS

There is wide agreement that psychiatric illness, including depression, involves CD of body temperature, mood, and sleep.[50,51] Moreover, acute sleep deprivation is effective in 40% to 60% of depressed subjects in improving mood within 24 to 48 hours, in contrast to antidepressant medications that typically require 2 to 8 weeks to have an effect.[52,53] The mechanisms underlying the mood-improving effects of this sudden acute circadian "shock" are as yet unknown, but suggest that directly manipulating the sleep-circadian system may be a pathway to explore. Along these lines, light (photic) therapy is another form of circadian manipulation that is effective in some depressed patients, and there are pharmaceutical agents for mood disorders, such as agomelatine, that interact with the melatonin system[54] as well as the use of melatonin itself for circadian phase shifting in seasonal affective disorder.[50]

Gross CDs, as measured by changes in sleep-activity cycles, are not the only rhythms that are perturbed in mood disorders. Psychotic major depression involves elevated evening cortisol levels, whereas the nonpsychotic form does not,[55] and elevated evening cortisol as well as CD are linked to metabolic syndrome.[56] Moreover, glucocorticoids are able to reset and synchronize the circadian clocks of peripheral tissues, including the liver, although the central pacemaker clock of the SCN does not respond to glucocorticoid.[24] Because almost every cell in the body expresses clock genes and glucocorticoid receptors are ubiquitous, the effects of CD can be profound: for example, in hamsters living in a light:dark cycle 2 hours different from the period of their normal clock, cardiac hypertrophy and renal failure are observed.[57]

NEURAL RESPONSES TO SLEEP DEPRIVATION

The brain is the master regulator of the neuroendocrine, autonomic, and immune systems. It is important to remember that it is also the master regulator of behaviors that contribute to unhealthy or healthy lifestyles, which, in turn, influence the physiologic processes of allostasis.[3] Therefore, chronic stress can therefore have direct and indirect effects on cumulative allostatic overload. There are many disparate changes driven by allostatic overload resulting from chronic stress. In animal models, chronic stress causes atrophy of neurons in the prefrontal cortex and hippocampus, brain regions involved in executive function, selective attention, and memory. On the other hand, chronic stress leads to hypertrophy of neurons in the amygdala, a region involved in fear, anxiety, and aggression.[58] Thus, chronic stress compromises the ability of an organism to learn, remember, and make decisions, as well as increases levels of anxiety and aggression.

Although not as much work has been conducted, it is obvious that the results of sleep deprivation, and perhaps to a lesser extent CD, share certain characteristics with chronic stress. For instance, there is recent evidence not only for cognitive impairment resulting from sleep restriction in animal models but also for altered levels of cytokines, oxidative stress markers, glycogen levels, and structural changes in the form of reduced dentate gyrus neurogenesis. Specifically, increases in brain levels of mRNA of the pro-inflammatory cytokine IL-1b are reported following sleep deprivation by gentle handling and is reported to be higher in daytime (during the normal sleep period in rodents) than in darkness (during the normal activity time for rodents).[59] Closely related to inflammatory processes, through the actions of NADPH oxidase,[60,61] is oxidative stress involving the generation of free radicals. Seventy-two hours of "flower pot" or platform sleep deprivation has been reported to increase oxidative stress in the mouse hippocampus, as measured by increased lipid peroxidation and increased ratios of oxidized to reduced glutathione.[62] Glycogen, found predominantly in white matter, is also profoundly affected by sleep deprivation and is reported to decrease by as much as 40% in rats deprived of sleep for 24 hours by novelty and gentle handling, an effect reversed by recovery sleep.[63,64] The specific consequences of this effect are not yet elucidated, although it is noteworthy that glycogen in astrocytes is able to sustain axon function during glucose deprivation in central nervous system white matter.[65]

With respect to memory and cognitive performance, there are numerous reports of impairments following sleep deprivation. For example, sleep deprivation by the platform (or flower pot) method leads to impaired performance of spatial memory in the Morris water maze,[66] and reduced CA1 hippocampal long-term potentiation.[67] Sleep deprivation using these methods also impairs retention of passive avoidance memory, a context-dependent, fear-memory task.[62] A different method of sleep deprivation, by gentle stimulation or novelty, following contextual fear conditioning impairs memory consolidation.[68] A 6-hour period of total sleep deprivation by novelty exposure impaired acquisition of a spatial task in the Morris water maze.[69] A 4-hour period of sleep deprivation by gentle stimulation impaired the late phase long term potentiation (LTP) in the dentate gyrus 48 hours later but had the opposite effect to enhance late-phase LTP in the prefrontal cortex.[70] Emotional behaviors are also affected by sleep deprivation. Increases in fighting behavior are observed following REM sleep deprivation[71]; there is also a report of increased aggression in the form of phencyclidine-induced muricide after sleep deprivation.[72,73] These findings harken to the results of increased aggression among cage mates in rats subjected to 21 days of 6h per day of chronic restraint stress during the resting period when some sleep deprivation may occur.[74] Thus, the effects of sleep deprivation are not simple and are influenced by their type, intensity, duration, and the types of behavioral outcomes measured.

The neural mechanisms of the effects of sleep deprivation on behavior are still not understood. However, sleep deprivation in rats using a treadmill for 96 hours has been reported to decrease proliferation of cells in the dentate gyrus of the hippocampal formation by as much as 50%.[75] A confound in this type of experiment is that the effects of activity are difficult to disentangle from the effects of the deprivation. A similar neural effect has also been reported by keeping rats in a slowly rotating drum, but, here again, there is a question of how much physical activity and physical stress may have contributed to the suppression of cell proliferation.[76] Nevertheless, sleep restriction by novelty exposure, a more subtle method, prevented the increased survival of new dentate gyrus neurons promoted by spatial training in a Morris water maze.[77] Recently, clear effects of sleep and sleep deprivation on hippocampal function has been demonstrated, showing that hippocampal network activity changes during sleep-dependent memory consolidation, and that sleep deprivation can affect hippocampal synaptic plasticity during defined timeframes.[78,79] Work in the visual cortex also shows that sleep affects memory consolidation,[80–82] suggesting these effects are not merely limited to the hippocampus.

INTEGRATION AND SUMMARY

Sleep is thought to be a neural state during which consolidation of declarative memories takes place.[83] Sleep deprivation, even for the course of the active period of the day in diurnal animals, increases the homeostatic drive to sleep, with resulting changes in pro-inflammatory cytokines and glycogen levels. Relatively brief deprivation of sleep promotes an exacerbation of these processes with progressively more severe physiologic, neurobiological, and behavioral consequences as the sleep deprivation is prolonged.

CD is a broader aspect of the problem of sleep disruption, with disruption of the circadian clock contributing to changes in sleep patterns, and sleep patterns potentially influencing the circadian clock. Shift work and jet lag are 2 common practices that have measurable effects on the brain and body.[84,85] For instance, long distance air travel with short turnaround has been reported to be associated with smaller volume of the temporal lobe and impaired performance on a visual-spatial cognitive task.[86]

The long-term consequences of sleep deprivation and CD constitute a form of allostatic load, with consequences involving hypertension, reduced parasympathetic tone, increased pro-inflammatory cytokines, increased oxidative stress, and increased evening cortisol and insulin. As noted above, reduced sleep and CD are associated with increased chances of cardiovascular disease and diabetes. Indeed, shorter sleep times have been associated with increased obesity.[44] Moreover, diabetes is associated with impaired hippocampal function,[87] decreased hippocampal volume,[88] and increased risk for Alzheimer disease[89,90], are observed.

In addition to the inflammatory and cardiometabolic changes that are observed, depressive illness is almost universally associated with disturbed sleep.[91] Thus, there are not only linkages between the multiple, interacting mediators that are involved in allostasis and allostatic load/overload, as summarized in **Fig. 1**, but also overlaps (ie, comorbidities) between disorders, such as diabetes, hypertension, cardiovascular disease, and depression, that are associated with excessive stress and with the dysregulation of the systems that normally promote allostasis and successful adaptation.

Sleep has important functions in maintaining homeostasis and sleep deprivation. Sleep deprivation or other forms of circadian disruption are stressors that have consequences for the brain as well as many body systems. Whether the sleep deprivation or circadian disruption is due to anxiety, depression, jetlag, shift work, or other aspects of a hectic lifestyle, there are consequences that contribute to allostatic load throughout the body. Taken together, these changes in brain and body

are further evidence that circadian disruption predisposes an individual to altered responses to stressors as well as impaired cognitive function and metabolic dysregulation. Sleep deprivation can be described as a chronic stressor that can cause allostatic overload, including mood and cognitive impairment and autonomic and metabolic dysregulation.

REFERENCES

1. Sterling P, Eyer J. Allostasis: a new paradigm to explain arousal pathology. In: Fisher S, Reason J, editors. Handbook of life stress, cognition and health. New York: John Wiley & Sons; 1988. p. 629–49.
2. McEwen BS, Stellar E. Stress and the individual: mechanisms leading to disease. Arch Intern Med 1993;153:2093–101.
3. McEwen BS. Protective and damaging effects of stress mediators. N Engl J Med 1998;338:171–9.
4. Munck A, Guyre PM. Glucocorticoids and immune function. In: Ader R, Felten DL, Cohen N, editors. Psychoneuroimmunology. San Diego (CA): Academic Press; 1991. p. 447–74.
5. Sapolsky RM. Physiological and pathophysiological implications of social stress in mammals. Coping with the environment: neural and endocrine mechanisms. New York: Oxford University Press; 2000. p. 517–32.
6. Borovikova LV, Ivanova S, Zhang M, et al. Vagus nerve stimulation attenuates the systemic inflammatory response to endotoxin. Nature 2000;405: 458–62.
7. Bierhaus A, Wolf J, Andrassy M, et al. A mechanism converting psychosocial stress into mononuclear cell activation. Proc Natl Acad Sci U S A 2003;100: 1920–5.
8. Sapolsky RM, Romero LM, Munck AU. How do glucocorticoids influence stress responses? Integrating permissive, suppressive, stimulatory, and preparative actions. Endocr Rev 2000;21:55–89.
9. McEwen BS, Wingfield JC. The concept of allostasis in biology and biomedicine. Horm Behav 2003; 43:2–15.
10. McEwen BS. Structural plasticity of the adult brain: how animal models help us understand brain changes in depression and systemic disorders related to depression. Dialogues Clin Neurosci 2004;6:119–33.
11. McEwen BS. Mood disorders and allostatic load. Biol Psychiatry 2003;54:200–7.
12. Sheline YI. Neuroimaging studies of mood disorder effects on the brain. Biol Psychiatry 2003;54:338–52.
13. Pitman RK. Hippocampal diminution in PTSD: more (or less?) than meets the eye. Hippocampus 2001; 11:73–4.

14. Bremner JD. Neuroimaging studies in post-traumatic stress disorder. Curr Psychiatry Rep 2002;4:254–63.

15. Butler MP, Kriegsfeld LJ, Silver R. Circadian regulation of endocrine functions. In: Pfaff D, Arnold A, Etgen A, et al, editors. Hormones, brain and behavior. 2nd edition. San Diego (CA): Academic Press; 2009. p. 473–505.

16. Cearley C, Churchill L, Krueger JM. Time of day differences in IL1beta and TNFalpha mRNA levels in specific regions of the rat brain. Neurosci Lett 2003;352:61–3.

17. Lange T, Dimitrov S, Born J. Effects of sleep and circadian rhythm on the human immune system. Ann N Y Acad Sci 2010;1193:48–59.

18. Jacobson L, Akana SF, Cascio CS, et al. Circadian variations in plasma corticosterone permit normal termination of adrenocorticotropin responses to stress. Endocrinology 1988;122:1343–8.

19. Boivin DB, Tremblay GM, James FO. Working on atypical schedules. Sleep Med 2007;8:578–89.

20. Knutsson A. Health disorders of shift workers. Occup Med (Lond) 2003;53:103–8.

21. Moore-Ede MC. Physiology of the circadian timing system: predictive versus reactive homeostasis. Am J Physiol 1986;250:R735–52.

22. Moore RY, Eichler VB. Loss of a circadian adrenal corticosterone rhythm following suprachiasmatic lesions in the rat. Brain Res 1972;42:201–6.

23. Klein DC, Moore RY, Reppert SM. Suprachiasmatic nucleus: the mind's clock. New York: Oxford University Press; 1991.

24. Balsalobre A, Brown SA, Marcacci L, et al. Resetting of circadian time in peripheral tissues by glucocorticoid signaling. Science 2000;289:2344–7.

25. Segall LA, Perrin JS, Walker CD, et al. Glucocorticoid rhythms control the rhythm of expression of the clock protein, Period2, in oval nucleus of the bed nucleus of the stria terminalis and central nucleus of the amygdala in rats. Neuroscience 2006;140:753–7.

26. Lamont EW, Robinson B, Stewart J, et al. The central and basolateral nuclei of the amygdala exhibit opposite diurnal rhythms of expression of the clock protein Period2. Proc Natl Acad Sci U S A 2005; 102:4180–4.

27. Karatsoreos IN, McEwen BS. Psychobiological allostasis: resistance, resilience and vulnerability. Trends Cogn Sci 2011;15:576–84.

28. Gilbertson MW, Paulus LA, Williston SK, et al. Neurocognitive function in monozygotic twins discordant for combat exposure: relationship to posttraumatic stress disorder. J Abnorm Psychol 2006;115:484–95.

29. Gilbertson MW, Shenton ME, Ciszewski A, et al. Smaller hippocampal volume predicts pathologic vulnerability to psychological trauma. Nat Neurosci 2002;5:1242–7.

30. Yoo SS, Gujar N, Hu P, et al. The human emotional brain without sleep–a prefrontal amygdala disconnect. Curr Biol 2007;17:R877–878.

31. Gianaros PJ, Jennings JR, Sheu LK, et al. Heightened functional neural activation to psychological stress covaries with exaggerated blood pressure reactivity. Hypertension 2007;49:134–40.

32. Gianaros PJ, Sheu LK. A review of neuroimaging studies of stressor-evoked blood pressure reactivity: emerging evidence for a brain-body pathway to coronary heart disease risk. Neuroimage 2009;47: 922–36.

33. Gianaros PJ, Sheu LK, Matthews KA, et al. Individual differences in stressor-evoked blood pressure reactivity vary with activation, volume, and functional connectivity of the amygdala. J Neurosci 2008;28:990–9.

34. Karatsoreos IN, Bhagat S, Bloss EB, et al. Disruption of circadian clocks has ramifications for metabolism, brain, and behavior. Proc Natl Acad Sci U S A 2011; 108:1657–62.

35. McEwen BS. Effects of adverse experiences for brain structure and function. Biol Psychiatry 2000; 48:721–31.

36. McEwen BS. Protective and damaging effects of stress mediators: central role of the brain. Dialogues Clin Neurosci 2006;8:367–81.

37. McEwen BS, Coirini H, Westlind-Danielsson A, et al. Steroid hormones as mediators of neural plasticity. J Steroid Biochem Mol Biol 1991;39:223–32.

38. Davis S, Mirick DK, Stevens RG. Night shift work, light at night, and risk of breast cancer. J Natl Cancer Inst 2001;93:1557–62.

39. Suwazono Y, Dochi M, Sakata K, et al. A longitudinal study on the effect of shift work on weight gain in male Japanese workers. Obesity (Silver Spring) 2008;16:1887–93.

40. Lowden A, Moreno C, Holmback U, et al. Eating and shift work - effects on habits, metabolism and performance. Scand J Work Environ Health 2010;36: 150–62.

41. Leproult R, Copinschi G, Buxton O, et al. Sleep loss results in an elevation of cortisol levels the next evening. Sleep 1997;20:865–70.

42. Spiegel K, Leproult R, Van Cauter E. Impact of sleep debt on metabolic and endocrine function. Lancet 1999;354:1435–9.

43. Spiegel K, Tasali E, Penev P, et al. Brief communication: sleep curtailment in healthy young men is associated with decreased leptin levels, elevated ghrelin levels, and increased hunger and appetite. Ann Intern Med 2004;141:846–50.

44. Gangwisch JE, Malaspina D, Boden-Albala B, et al. Inadequate sleep as a risk factor for obesity: analyses of the NHANES I. Sleep 2005;28:1289–96.

45. Matthews KA, Dahl RE, Owens JF, et al. Sleep duration and insulin resistance in healthy black and white adolescents. Sleep 2012;35:1353–8.

46. St-Onge MP, O'Keeffe M, Roberts AL, et al. Short sleep duration, glucose dysregulation and hormonal regulation of appetite in men and women. Sleep 2012;35:1503–10.

47. Vetrivelan R, Fuller PM, Yokota S, et al. Metabolic effects of chronic sleep restriction in rats. Sleep 2012;35:1511–20.

48. Vgontzas AN, Zoumakis E, Bixler EO, et al. Adverse effects of modest sleep restriction on sleepiness, performance, and inflammatory cytokines. J Clin Endocrinol Metab 2004;89:2119–26.

49. Friedman EM, Hayney MS, Love GD, et al. Social relationships, sleep quality, and interleukin-6 in aging women. Proc Natl Acad Sci U S A 2005;102:18757–62.

50. Lewy AJ, Lefler BJ, Emens JS, et al. The circadian basis of winter depression. Proc Natl Acad Sci U S A 2006;103:7414–9.

51. Karatsoreos IN. Links between circadian rhythms and psychiatric disease. Front Behav Neurosci 2014;8:162.

52. Vogel GW, Thompson FC Jr, Thurmond A, et al. The effect of REM deprivation on depression. Psychosomatics 1973;14:104–7.

53. Wirz-Justice A, Van den Hoofdakker RH. Sleep deprivation in depression: what do we know, where do we go? Biol Psychiatry 1999;46:445–53.

54. Morley-Fletcher S, Mairesse J, Soumier A, et al. Chronic agomelatine treatment corrects behavioral, cellular, and biochemical abnormalities induced by prenatal stress in rats. Psychopharmacology 2011;217:301–13.

55. Keller J, Flores B, Gomez RG, et al. Cortisol circadian rhythm alterations in psychotic major depression. Biol Psychiatry 2006;60:275–81.

56. Rintamaki R, Grimaldi S, Englund A, et al. Seasonal changes in mood and behavior are linked to metabolic syndrome. PLoS One 2008;3:e1482.

57. Martino TA, Oudit GY, Herzenberg AM, et al. Circadian rhythm disorganization produces profound cardiovascular and renal disease in hamsters. Am J Physiol Regul Integr Comp Physiol 2008;294:R1675–83.

58. McEwen BS, Chattarji S. Molecular mechanisms of neuroplasticity and pharmacological implications: the example of tianeptine. Eur Neuropsychopharmacol 2004;14:S497–502.

59. Taishi P, Chen Z, Obal FJ, et al. Sleep-associated changes in interleukin-1beta mRNA in the brain. J Interferon Cytokine Res 1998;18:793–8.

60. Clark RA, Valente AJ. Nuclear factor kappa B activation by NADPH oxidases. Mech Ageing Dev 2004;125:799–810.

61. Tang J, Liu J, Zhou C, et al. Role of NADPH oxidase in the brain injury of intracerebral hemorrhage. J Neurochem 2005;94:1342–50.

62. Silva RH, Abilio VC, Takatsu AL, et al. Role of hippocampal oxidative stress in memory deficits induced by sleep deprivation in mice. Neuropharmacology 2004;46:895–903.

63. Kong J, Shepel PN, Holden CP, et al. Brain glycogen decreases with increased periods to wakefulness: implications for homeostatic drive to sleep. J Neurosci 2002;22:5581–7.

64. Brown AM. Brain glycogen re-awakened. J Neurochem 2004;89:537–52.

65. Wender R, Brown AM, Fern R, et al. Astrocytic glycogen influences axon function and survival during glucose deprivation in central white matter. J Neurosci 2000;20:6804–10.

66. Youngblood BD, Zhou J, Smagin GN, et al. Sleep deprivation by the "flower pot" technique and spatial reference memory. Physiol Behav 1997;61:249–56.

67. Kim EY, Mahmoud GS, Grover LM. REM sleep deprivation inhibits LTP in vivo in area CA1 of rat hippocampus. Neurosci Lett 2005;388:163–7.

68. Graves LA, Heller EA, Pack AI, et al. Sleep deprivation selectively impairs memory consolidation for contextual fear conditioning. Learn Mem 2003;10:168–76.

69. Guan Z, Peng X, Fang J. Sleep deprivation impairs spatial memory and decreases extracellular signal-regulated kinase phosphorylation in the hippocampus. Brain Res 2004;1018:38–47.

70. Romcy-Pereira R, Pavlides C. Distinct modulatory effects of sleep on the maintenance of hippocampal and medial prefrontal cortex LTP. Eur J Neurosci 2004;20:3453–62.

71. de Paula HM, Hoshino K. Correlation between the fighting rates of REM sleep-deprived rats and susceptibility to the 'wild running' of audiogenic seizures. Brain Res 2002;926:80–5.

72. Musty RE, Consroe PF. Phencyclidine produces aggressive behavior in rapid eye movement sleep-deprived rats. Life Sci 1982;30:1733–8.

73. Russell JW, Singer G. Relations between muricide, circadian rhythm and consummatory behavior. Physiol Behav 1983;30:23–7.

74. Wood GE, Young LT, Reagan LP, et al. Acute and chronic restraint stress alter the incidence of social conflict in male rats. Horm Behav 2003;43:205–13.

75. Guzman-Marin R, Suntsova N, Stewart DR, et al. Sleep deprivation reduces proliferation of cells in the dentate gyrus of the hippocampus in rats. J Physiol 2003;549(2):563–71.

76. Roman V, Van der Borght K, Leemburg SA, et al. Sleep restriction by forced activity reduces hippocampal cell proliferation. Brain Res 2005;1065:53–9.

77. Hairston IS, Little MT, Scanlon MD, et al. Sleep restriction suppresses neurogenesis induced by hippocampus-dependent learning. J Neurophysiol 2005;94:4224–33.

78. Prince TM, Wimmer M, Choi J, et al. Sleep deprivation during a specific 3-hour time window post-training

impairs hippocampal synaptic plasticity and memory. Neurobiol Learn Mem 2014;109:122–30.

79. Ognjanovski N, Maruyama D, Lashner N, et al. CA1 hippocampal network activity changes during sleep-dependent memory consolidation. Front Syst Neurosci 2014;8:61.

80. Aton SJ, Seibt J, Dumoulin M, et al. Mechanisms of sleep-dependent consolidation of cortical plasticity. Neuron 2009;61:454–66.

81. Aton SJ, Broussard C, Dumoulin M, et al. Visual experience and subsequent sleep induce sequential plastic changes in putative inhibitory and excitatory cortical neurons. Proc Natl Acad Sci U S A 2013;110:3101–6.

82. Aton SJ, Suresh A, Broussard C, et al. Sleep promotes cortical response potentiation following visual experience. Sleep 2014;37:1163–70.

83. Gais S, Born J. Declarative memory consolidation: mechanisms acting during human sleep. Learn Mem 2004;11:679–85.

84. Atkinson G, Davenne D. Relationships between sleep, physical activity and human health. Physiol Behav 2007;90:229–36.

85. Karlson B, Eek FC, Hansen AM, et al. Diurnal cortisol pattern of shift workers on workday and a day off. Scand J Work Environ Health 2006;Suppl (2):27–34.

86. Cho K. Chronic 'jet lag' produces temporal lobe atrophy and spatial cognitive deficits. Nat Neurosci 2001;4:567–8.

87. Hendrickx H, McEwen BS, van der Ouderaa F. Metabolism, mood and cognition in aging: the importance of lifestyle and dietary intervention. Neurobiol Aging 2005;26S:S1–5.

88. Gold SM, Dziobek I, Sweat V, et al. Hippocampal damage and memory impairments as possible early brain complications of type 2 diabetes. Diabetologia 2007;50:711–9.

89. Arvanitakis Z, Wilson RS, Bienias JL, et al. Diabetes mellitus and risk of Alzheimer disease and decline in cognitive function. Arch Neurol 2004; 61:661–6.

90. Rasgon N, Jarvik L. Insulin resistance, affective disorders, and Alzheimer's disease: review and hypothesis. J Gerontol 2004;59A:178–83.

91. Tsuno N, Besset A, Ritchie K. Sleep and depression. J Clin Psychiatry 2005;66:1254–69.

Sleep in the Context of Healthy Aging and Psychiatric Syndromes

Daniel B. Kay, PhD[a],*, Joseph M. Dzierzewski, PhD[b,c]

KEYWORDS

- Sleep • Aging • Psychiatric disorders

KEY POINTS

- Sleep disturbances in the context of psychiatric conditions in late-life creates an ambiguous and challenging scenario for researchers and clinicians.
- Investigations of the potential shared biological substrates between sleep disorders and psychiatric conditions in late-life and randomized, controlled trials aimed at improving the sleep of older adults with concurrent psychiatric conditions are lacking.
- An important caveat regarding treatment is that it may be difficult on occasion to determine the best treatment plan for sleep disorders in the context of psychiatric conditions in late-life.
- The modal treatment for sleep disorders in the context of psychiatric conditions in late-life is medication.
- Cognitive-behavioral therapy is an evidence-based treatment for sleep disorders and should be the treatment of choice, even in the context of conditions thought to be biologic and/or psychiatric.

INTRODUCTION

Humans spend approximately one-third of their lives asleep. Whether due to evolutionary or ontogenetic factors, sleep and psychiatric disorders change with age. Although much of sleep remains an enigma, the field of sleep medicine is experiencing an exponential increase in its understanding of the causes, correlates, and consequences of sleep disturbances. Although the relationship between age-related sleep and psychiatric conditions is a common clinical observation, empirical investigations into these associations remain scarce. Thus, treating patients with symptoms of sleep disorders in the context of psychiatric conditions remains a major challenge. This article reviews the state-of-the-science of sleep disorders in the context of psychiatric conditions in late-life.

SLEEP IN AGING

Both self-report and polysomnographic (PSG) studies of sleep document age-related changes in sleep architecture. Subjective sleep quality decreases with age. Shortened and less restorative sleep, more frequent nighttime awakenings (NTA), increased time awake in the night, and early morning awakenings[1] are well documented with aging. Sleep is "structurally lighter" in the elderly. Cross-sectional studies using PSGs have shown that older adults spend less time in deep, slow-wave sleep (SWS), spend more time in the light, nonrestorative stages 1 and 2 sleep, and experience more frequent shifts from one sleep stage to another. These studies show more frequent arousals, shorter rapid eye movement (REM) sleep latencies, more and longer periods of α (wake)

Funding sources: Daniel B. Kay, PhD was support by T32 training grants (HL082610, PI: Daniel J. Buysse, MD and AG020499, PI: Michael Marsiski, PhD). Joseph M Dzierzewski, PhD was supported by UCLA Claude Pepper Center (5P30AG028748), UCLA CTSI (UL1TR000124), and VA Advanced Geriatrics Fellowship.
^a Department of Psychiatry, University of Pittsburgh, Pittsburgh; ^b David Geffen School of Medicine, University of California, Los Angeles, California; ^c Geriatric Research, Education, and Clinical Center, VA Greater Los Angeles Healthcare System, Los Angeles, California
* Corresponding author.
E-mail address: DBK16@pitt.edu

Sleep Med Clin 10 (2015) 11–15
http://dx.doi.org/10.1016/j.jsmc.2014.11.012
1556-407X/15/$ – see front matter
© 2015 Elsevier Inc. All rights reserved.

activity during sleep, and a lower awakening threshold in the elderly.[1-3] Sleep efficiency is the only parameter that declines significantly after the age of 60.[4] A meta-analysis of age-related sleep changes shows that increased age is associated with extended sleep onset latency (SOL), increased wake after sleep onset (WASO), more NTA, and decreased total sleep time (TST).[5] Interestingly, objectively measured WASO, NTA, and TST correlate more with age than self-report.

Night-to-night inconsistency, or intraindividual variability, increases in older adults with and without sleep complaints, both objectively and subjectively.[6,7] Importantly, although on average subjective and objective measures of sleep decline with age, self-report and PSG measures correlate poorly on a night-to-night basis.[8]

POOR SLEEP IN LATE-LIFE

Epidemiologic estimates suggest that as many as 65% of older adults complain about at least one of several sleep disturbances.[9] Poor sleep in the elderly relates to higher mental and physical morbidity, hospitalizations, mortality, and suicidality (reviewed in[1]). The most common complaints include frequent awakenings during the night, waking too early, and difficulty falling asleep.[9] Of these, late-life insomnia is among the most costly and preventable health problems in the United States. The diagnosis of insomnia disorder is based on a complaint of chronic (>3 months) difficulty initiating or maintaining sleep, or unrefreshing sleep occurring at least 3 nights per week.[10,11] Although insomnia is not part of normal aging, the incidence, prevalence, severity, and chronicity of it increase with age.

Because of considerable interindividual variability in late-life sleep, insomnia and normal age-related changes overlap, as do their consequences on daytime functioning. Older adults experience similar sleep very differently. For example, in late-life, women are more likely than men to complain of insomnia, although objective sleep architecture is generally more disturbed in men.[12] Notably, although aging is more correlated with objective measures of sleep architecture, subjective measures are more predictive of insomnia and its associated social costs and personal mental/physical sequelae.

SLEEP AND OTHER CONDITIONS: PRIMARY VERSUS SECONDARY

The prevalence rate of sleep complaints among older adults drops to as low as ~2% after eliminating all who complain of a comorbid mental/

physical condition.[13] However, calculating prevalence rates after controlling for potential comorbid conditions should be viewed with caution, because co-occurrence does not negate independence. Approximately 7 of 8 older adults who report sleep disturbances report at least one other major mental/psychological disorder, particularly depression, heart disease, pain, and memory problems.[14] Such co-occurrences have traditionally led to 2 unsupported conclusions: (1) sleep disturbances are merely symptoms of mental/psychological disorders that cannot be improved without successful treatment of the primary condition and (2) sleep problems will subside with the successful treatment of the primary condition. Although in some instances this may be true, clinical research suggests that sleep disturbances are treatable even in the context of a severe medical problem (reviewed in[1]). Sleep complaints persist in most patients following treatment of their primary medical or psychological condition.[15] Nevertheless, the vast majority of clinicians and patients think that poor sleep is inextricably tied to another underlying pathologic condition.

To counteract this bias, the National Institutes of Health issued a statement in 2005 recommending that disturbed sleep no longer be routinely conceptualized as secondary to another disorder.[16]

SLEEP AND PSYCHIATRIC CONDITIONS

Across the lifespan, poor sleep is often comorbid with psychiatric disorders. More than 30% of older individuals with insomnia have an accompanying psychiatric disorder (reviewed in[1]) The relationship between sleep and mental health has long been recognized. In 1867, Wilhelm Griesinger[17] outlined 4 major psychological conditions highly correlated with sleep disturbance: depression, hypochondriasis, mania, and psychosis. The basic relationship between depression, anxiety, mania, psychosis, and sleep disturbances remains a robust finding. This article reviews the relationship between age-related changes in sleep and the aforementioned mental health problems, with the addition of a brief discussion on dementia. Although the specificity of a sleep disturbance as psychiatrically diagnostic is low,[1] understanding this relationship enriches the understanding of both.

Depression

Approximately 14% of older adults in the United States experience significant symptoms of depression.[18] About one-quarter of these meet criteria for major depressive disorder, among the highest incidence of any major psychiatric disorder. Clinical and epidemiologic evidence indicate that depression shares a robust relationship with sleep disturbances and that this relationship is likely bidirectional. In a general population, sleep disturbance is present in about 60% of depressed individuals. It is one of the most common symptoms of mild depression.[19] Several of the changes that occur with sleep in depression resemble sleep changes that also occur with aging, specifically, reduced sleep length, reduced sleep continuity, decreased REM sleep latency, and a decline in sleep depth.[20] These age-related changes in sleep are more severe in older adults with depression compared with healthy older adults.[21]

In older adults, depressive symptoms frequently appear with severe insomnia, both the sleep-onset and the sleep-maintenance varieties.[22] Early morning awakenings are the most frequent sleep disturbance in conjunction with late-life depression.[23,24] Insomnia in conjunction with depression has a poorer prognosis than depression alone and predicts future major depressive episodes.[25,26] Targeted assessment and treatment of comorbid insomnia in late-life depression are indicated.

Mania

The 3-year incidence of bipolar disorders in adults over the age of 55 is among the lowest of all DSM-IV disorders (bipolar I = 0.54%, bipolar II = 0.34%[27]). Bipolar disorder deserves consideration because of its substantial personal and social burden. There is an absolute dearth of research on the relationship between age-related changes in sleep and mania. In younger samples, decreases in self-reported sleep duration commonly precede a manic episode.[28] Objective sleep changes in bipolar disorder include abnormalities in REM latency, duration, and density (reviewed in[29]). Increased SWS is predictive of manic symptoms and impairment at 3 months, whereas greater time spent in stage 2 sleep is predictive of lower levels of manic symptoms and impairment. Clozapine (commonly prescribed to treat resistant mania) increases time spent in stage 2 sleep,[30] suggesting that stage 2 sleep contributes to countering mania. Research in this area is warranted.

Anxiety

Anxiety is a common problem in late-life. The 3-year incidence of anxiety disorders in adults over the age of 60 ranges from 0.58% (social phobia) to 1.63% (generalized anxiety disorder; GAD[27]). Although the prevalence of anxiety disorders decreases with age, there is evidence that this may be a research artifact because of (1) cohort effects (ie, older adults may be less likely to report anxiety symptoms), (2) differences in

how anxiety is experienced with the aged and how it is measured by researchers (ie, more subclinical anxiety in late-life and decreased physiologic reactivity), and/or (3) sampling bias. Anxiety disorders in late-life, especially GAD, are highly associated with sleep disturbances even when controlling for comorbid depression. About one-half of older adults with an anxiety disorder also have sleep disturbance, most commonly sleep-onset difficulties.[23] Among patients with anxiety, the degree of sleep disturbance correlates with anxiety severity.[4] Sleep disturbances in late-life GAD are more severe than in younger GAD patients.[31] The high comorbidity of sleep and anxiety may be related to the fact that anxiety in most everyone, syndromic or not, typically disrupts sleep, briefly or over an extended time frame (reviewed in[32]).

Treating older adults with comorbid insomnia and anxiety can be challenging. Cognitive behavioral therapy (CBT) of comorbid anxiety or insomnia may be effective in treating the anxiety. However, treating one may not result in improvement in the other.[33] Combining components of CBT for anxiety and insomnia may effectively address both, but is not yet supported by research.[32]

Psychosis

Sleep complaints are common with schizophrenia in late-life and are more severe than in normal aging.[34] Sleep abnormalities occur in both medicated and unmediated patients. In younger patients, schizophrenia is related to reduced sleep length, longer sleep latencies, and poorer sleep efficiency.[35] In late-life, schizophrenia is related to increased time in bed, TST, more night-time awakenings, greater WASO, and more and longer naps.[34] These sleep disturbances may be due to the disorder. Conversely, changes in sleep can exacerbate symptoms and are predictive of psychotic episodes, including psychotic symptoms, impairments in cognitive functioning, negative symptoms, and poor quality of life.[36] Little research exists.

Dementia

The term dementia loosely describes symptoms dominated by negative cognitive changes, such as declines in memory, attention, executive functions, and language in the presence of significant functional impairment in activities of daily living, such as self-care and bowel/bladder management. Dementia is not a disorder, but rather a symptom of several dementing conditions (Alzheimer disease [AD], Parkinson disease, Lewy body disease). Because dementia results from different neurologic and pathologic abnormalities, sleep presentation differs considerably from condition to condition.

AD, the single most prevalent dementing disorder, is the focus of this section. Many untoward changes in sleep occur in AD. Both wake and sleep electroencephalography show a general slowing of waveforms. The sleep of AD patients is less efficient and shows more time in lighter sleep, less time in deep sleep, a decrease in time in REM sleep, and more arousals than controls.[37] A rather disruptive problem is "sundowning," which refers to AD patients' propensity to become more agitated, active, and confused during the evening hours. Sundowning is a predictor of institutionalization. Treatments of sleep disturbances in AD patients are underdeveloped and lack consensus. Because sleep problems associated AD patients are generally viewed as multifactorial, potential treatments should be individually tailored and both the causes of the disturbance and the context in which the disturbance occurs should be considered (for a review, see[38]). This area lacks research.

SUMMARY

Sleep disturbances in the context of psychiatric conditions in late-life create an ambiguous and challenging scenario for researchers and clinicians. Important research agenda and treatment implications abound. Investigations of the potential shared biological substrates between sleep disorders and psychiatric conditions in late-life and randomized, controlled trials aimed at improving the sleep of older adults with concurrent psychiatric conditions are lacking. An important caveat regarding treatment is that it may be difficult on occasion to determine the best treatment plan for sleep disorders in the context of psychiatric conditions in late-life. When comorbid with another condition, sleep complaints deserve focused assessment and treatment. The modal treatment of sleep disorders in the context of psychiatric conditions in late-life is medication. Because of concerns of polypharmacy, drug interactions, and differing metabolisms in late-life, pharmaceutical interventions should be used sparingly.[39] Cognitive-behavioral therapy is an evidence-based treatment for sleep disorders and should be the treatment of choice, even in the context of conditions thought to be biological and/or psychiatric.

REFERENCES

1. Morgan K. Sleep and aging. In: Lichstein KL, Morin CM, editors. Treatment of late-life insomnia. Thousand Oaks (CA): Sage; 2000. p. 3–36.

2. Boselli M, Parrino L, Smerieri A, et al. Effect of age on EEG arousals in normal sleep. Sleep 1998;21: 361–7.

3. Zepelin H, McDonald CS, Zammit GK. Effects of age on auditory awakening thresholds. J Gerontol 1984; 39:294–300.

4. Ohayon MM, Carskadon MA, Guilleminault C, et al. Meta-analysis of quantitative sleep parameters from childhood to old age in healthy individuals: developing normative sleep values across the human lifespan. Sleep 2004;27:1255–73.

5. Floyd JA, Medler SM, Ager JW, et al. Age-related changes in initiation and maintenance of sleep: a meta-analysis. Res Nurs Health 2000;23:106–17.

6. Buysse DJ, Cheng Y, Germain A, et al. Night-to-night sleep variability in older adults with and without chronic insomnia. Sleep Med 2010;11:56–64.

7. Dzierzewski JM, McCrae CS, Rowe M, et al. Nightly sleep patterns in older adults: night-to-night fluctuations in the sleep of older good-noncomplaining, good-complaining, poor-noncomplaining, poor-complaining/insomnia, and caregivers. Sleep 2008;31: A104.

8. Kay DB, Dzierzewski JM, Rowe M, et al. Greater night-to-night variability in sleep discrepancy among older adults with a sleep complaint compared to noncomplaining older adults. Behav Sleep Med 2013;11:76–90.

9. Newman AB, Enright PL, Manolio TA, et al. Sleep disturbance, psychological correlates, and cardiovascular disease in 5201 older adults: the Cardiovascular Health Study. J Am Geriatr Soc 1997;45: 1–7.

10. International Classification of Sleep Disorders. 3rd ed. Darien, IL: American Academy of Sleep Medicine; 2014.

11. American Psychiatric Association. Diagnostic and Statistical Manual of Mental Disorders. 5th ed. Arlington, VA: American Psychiatric Association; 2013.

12. Vitiello MV, Larsen LH, Moe KE. Age-related sleep change gender and estrogen effects on the subjective-objective sleep quality relationship of healthy, noncomplaining older men and women. J Psychosom Res 2004;56:503–10.

13. Vitiello MV, Moe KE, Prinz PN. Sleep complaints cosegregate with illness in older adults: clinical research informed by and informing epidemiological studies of sleep. J Psychosom Res 2002;53: 555–9.

14. Foley D, Ancoli-Israel S, Britz P, et al. Sleep disturbance and chronic disease in older adults: results of the 2003 National Sleep Foundation Sleep in America survey. J Psychosom Res 2004;56:497–502.

15. Nierenberg AA, Keefe BR, Leslie VC, et al. Residual symptoms in depressed patients who respond acutely to fluoxetine. J Clin Psychiatry 1999;60:221–5.

16. NIH State-of-the-Science Conference Statement on manifestations and management of chronic insomnia in adults. NIH Consens State Sci Statements 2005; 22:1–30.

17. Griesinger W. Mental pathology and therapeutics. 1867. Available at: http://books.google.com/books/reader?id=SVZHAAAAYAAJ&printsec=frontcover&output=reader. Accessed June 18, 2011.

18. Zivin K, Llewellyn DJ, Lang IA, et al. Depression among older adults in the United States and England. Am J Geriatr Psychiatry 2010;18:1036–44.

19. Carragher N, Mewton L, Slade T, et al. An item response analysis of the DSM-IV criteria for major depression: findings from the Australian National Survey of Mental Health and Wellbeing. J Affect Disord 2011;130:92–8.

20. Kupfer DJ, Reynolds CF 3rd, Ulrich RF, et al. EEG sleep, depression, and aging. Neurobiol Aging 1982;3:351–60.

21. Knowles JB, MacLean AW. Age related changes in sleep in depressed and healthy subjects: a meta-analysis. Neuropsychopharmacology 1990;3:251–9.

22. Maggi S, Langlois JA, Minicuci N, et al. Sleep complaints in community-dwelling older persons: prevalence, associated factors, and reported causes. J Am Geriatr Soc 1998;46:161–8.

23. Mallon L, Broman J-E, Hetta J. Sleep difficulties in relation to depression and anxiety in elderly adults. Nord J Psychiatry 2000b;54:355–60.

24. Rodin J, McAvay G, Timko C. A longitudinal study of depressed mood and sleep disturbances in elderly adults. J Gerontol 1988;43:45–53.

25. Roberts RE, Shema SJ, Kaplan GA, et al. Sleep complaints and depression in an aging cohort: a prospective perspective. Am J Psychiatry 2000; 157:81–8.

26. Mallon L, Broman JE, Hetta J. Relationship between insomnia, depression, and mortality: a 12-year follow-up of older adults in the community. Int Psychogeriatr 2000a;12:295–306.

27. Chou K-L, Mackenzie CS, Liang K, et al. Three-year incidence and predators of first-onset DSM-IV mood, anxiety, and substance use disorders in older adults: results from wave 2 of the National Epidemiological Survey on Alcohol and Related Conditions. J Clin Psychiatry 2011;72:144–55.

28. Jackson A, Cavanagh J, Scott J. A systematic review of manic and depressive prodromes. J Affect Disord 2003;74:209–17.

29. Eidelman P, Talbot LS, Gruber J, et al. Sleep architecture as correlate and predictor of symptoms and impairment in inter-episode bipolar disorder: taking on the challenge of medication effects. J Sleep Res 2010;19:516–24.

30. Hinze-Selch D, Mullington J, Orth A, et al. Effects of clozapine on sleep: a longitudinal study. Biol Psychiatry 1997;42:260–6.

31. Brenes GA, Miller ME, Stanley MA, et al. Insomnia in older adults with generalized anxiety disorder. Am J Geriatr Psychiatry 2009;17:465–72.

32. Magee JC, Carmin CN. The relationship between sleep and anxiety in older adults. Curr Psychiatry Rep 2010;12:13–9.

33. Rybarczyk B, Lopez M, Alsten C, et al. Efficacy of two behavioral treatment programs for comorbid insomnia. Psychol Aging 2002;17:288–98.

34. Martin JL, Jeste DV, Ancoli-Israel S. Older schizophrenia patients have more disrupted sleep and circadian rhythms than age-matched comparison subjects. J Psychiatr Res 2005;39:251–9.

35. Benca RM, Obermeyer WH, Thisted RA, et al. Sleep and psychiatric disorders: a meta-analysis. Arch Gen Psychiatry 1992;49:651–70.

36. Martin J, Jeste DV, Caligiuri MP, et al. Actigraphic estimates of circadian rhythms and sleep/wake in older schizophrenia patients. Schizophr Res 2001;47:77–86.

37. Bliwise DL. Sleep in normal aging and dementia. Sleep 1993;16:40–81.

38. McCurry SM, Reynolds CF, Ancoli-Isreal S, et al. Treatment of sleep disturbance in Alzheimer's disease. Sleep Med Rev 2000;4:603–28.

39. Dzierzewski JM, O'Brien EM, Kay D, et al. Tackling sleeplessness: psychological treatment options for insomnia in older adults. Nat Sci Sleep 2010;2:47–61.

Sleep Disturbances in Depression

Michael J. Murphy, MD, PhD[a,b], Michael J. Peterson, MD, PhD[c,d],*

KEYWORDS

- Sleep • Major depressive disorder • Insomnia • Hypersomnia • Cognitive behavioral therapy
- Hypnotic • Antidepressant

KEY POINTS

- Major depressive disorder is frequently accompanied by subjective sleep disturbances and polysomnographic abnormalities.
- Residual sleep disturbance after a major depressive episode is linked to future relapses.
- Sleep problems may be the first sign of the onset of a major depressive episode.
- Obstructive sleep apnea may mimic major depressive disorder and increase risk for depression.
- Pharmacotherapy or behavioral approaches are useful in depressed patients with sleep disturbances.

MAJOR DEPRESSIVE DISORDER
Epidemiology and Comorbidity

Major depressive disorder is one of the most common psychiatric illnesses in the United States, with an estimated lifetime prevalence of up to 17%.[1] Affected individuals are at high risk for comorbid medical and psychiatric illness and have worse medical outcomes than the general population.[2,3] Major depressive disorder is highly correlated with suicidality, and up to 3% of affected individuals ultimately complete suicide.[3] The societal cost of major depressive disorder is massive; according to some estimates it may be responsible for up to $44 billion a year in lost productivity in the United States alone.[4] Several pharmacologic agents have been developed to treat depression including multiple classes of antidepressant medications (**Table 1**). These drugs, even when combined with psychotherapy, will ultimately fail in approximately one-third of patients.[5] Furthermore, treatment for major depressive disorder typically takes at least several weeks to produce noticeable effects.[5]

Diagnosis

Major depressive episodes are defined by a history of a 2 weeks or longer of depressed mood or anhedonia (diminished enjoyment of normally pleasurable activities) with at least 3 of the following: significant weight change or change in appetite, psychomotor agitation or retardation, feelings of worthlessness or guilt, diminished ability to concentrate, recurrent thoughts of death (or suicidal ideation or suicide attempts), and insomnia or hypersomnia.[6] There are several subtypes and modifiers of depression, each defined by a distinctive set of clinical features and typically responsive to specific types of treatments. Atypical depression, characterized by mood reactivity, hyperphagia, hypersomnia, and hypersensitivity to interpersonal rejection, is described as responding well to monoamine oxidase inhibitors and poorly to tricyclic antidepressants.[6] Patients with melancholic depression show terminal insomnia, weight loss, and ruminate on negative thoughts and are more likely to respond positively to sleep deprivation

[a] Department of Psychiatry, Massachusetts General Hospital, 55 Fruit Street, Boston, MA 02114, USA; [b] McLean Hospital, 115 Mill Street, Belmont, MA 02478, USA; [c] Department of Psychiatry, University of Wisconsin School of Medicine and Public Health, 6001 Research Park Boulevard, Madison, WI 53719, USA; [d] Department of Psychiatry, University of Wisconsin School of Medicine and Public Health, B6/593 Clinical Science Center, 600 Highland Avenue, Madison, WI 53792, USA
* Corresponding author.
E-mail address: mpeterson2@wisc.edu

Sleep Med Clin 10 (2015) 17–23
http://dx.doi.org/10.1016/j.jsmc.2014.11.009
1556-407X/15/$ – see front matter © 2015 Elsevier Inc. All rights reserved.

Table 1
Antidepressant effects on sleep

Medication Class Examples	Dosage: Depression (Insomnia[a])	Pharmacologic Mechanism	Effects on Sleep
Tricyclic antidepressants			
Amitriptyline(Elavil)	75–150 mg (25–50 mg)	Inhibit serotonin and norepinephrine reuptake Anticholinergic and antihistaminergic effects	Sedation REM sleep suppression Increased stage 2 sleep
Nortriptyline (Pamelor)	50–150 mg (25–50 mg)		
Doxepin (Sinequan)	75–300 mg (6–50 mg)		
Clomipramine (Anafranil)	100–250 mg		
MAOis			
Phenelzine(Nardil)	45–90 mg	Inhibit monoamine oxidase, thus increasing norepinephrine, serotonin, and dopamine	Insomnia Potent REM suppression
Tranylcypromine(Parnate)	30–60 mg		
Serotonin reuptake inhibitors			
Fluoxetine (Prozac)	20–80 mg	Inhibit serotonin reuptake	Insomnia REM suppression Increased eye movements in NREM sleep
Sertraline (Zoloft)	50–200 mg		
Paroxetine (Paxil)	15–60 mg		
Citalopam (Celexa)	20–40 mg		
Escitalopram (Lexapro)	10–30 mg		
Serotonin-norepinephrine reuptake inhibitors			
Venlafaxine (Effexor)	150–450 mg	Inhibit serotonin and norepinephrine reuptake	Insomnia REM suppression Increased eye movements in NREM sleep
Duloxetine (Cymbalta)	20–120 mg		
Other antidepressants:			
Trazodone (Desyrel)	150–600 mg (25–75 mg)	Inhibit serotonin reuptake. Blocks alpha1 adrenoreceptors Serotonin-2 A receptor antagonist	Sedation
Bupropion (Wellbutrin)	100–450 mg	Inhibits norepinephrine and dopamine reuptake	Insomnia/activation
Mirtazapine (Remeron)	15–45 mg (7.5–15 mg)	Alpha2 receptor antagonist. Serotonin-2 and -3 receptor antagonist. Antihistaminergic	Sedation, REM sleep suppression

[a] Use of these medications for treatment of insomnia is an off-label usage, not approved by the US Food and Drug Administration.

(see later discussion). In addition, some depressed individuals can develop psychotic symptoms such as delusions and hallucinations and the recommended treatment includes antipsychotics in addition to antidepressant medication.[6] In major depressive disorder with a seasonal pattern (also known colloquially as seasonal affective disorder), there is a recurrent pattern of depressive episodes that reliably occur during the same time of year (usually winter) for at least 2 consecutive years. Seasonal affective disorder can be treated with light therapy in addition to medications and psychotherapy.[6]

Sleep and Depression

One of the most consistent symptoms associated with major depressive disorder is sleep disturbance.[7–9] These problems with sleep regulation are not secondary to the illness; rather, they often precede the depressive episodes and can persist during remission. Improving sleep in depressed patients is found to improve outcomes.[10,11] In addition, imposed sleep deprivation can precipitate depressive episodes in susceptible individuals and alleviate depressive symptoms in others.[7] These observations dictate that practitioners of sleep medicine are aware of patients with major depressive disorder and alert to the importance of addressing sleep complaints in this population.

BIOCHEMICAL PATHWAYS UNDERLYING MOOD AND SLEEP
Monoamines

Although the precise physiologic correlates of sleep and mood are only partially understood, a growing body of biochemical evidence suggests that the mechanisms that control sleep overlap with the mechanisms that regulate mood. The transition into rapid-eye-movement (REM) sleep is accompanied by a rapid decrease in monoaminergic (serotonin, norepinephrine, and dopamine) tone and a concomitant increase in cholinergic tone.[12] It is hypothesized that dysregulation of these same monoamine neurotransmitters is related to major depressive disorder and, therefore, may be responsible for the REM sleep abnormalities noted in patients with major depressive disorder.[7] In fact, most commonly prescribed antidepressant medications act to increase monoaminergic tone and reduce REM sleep. However, one caveat is that some of these drugs can improve mood symptoms while leaving REM sleep unchanged. Furthermore, other effective antidepressant medications do not increase monoaminergic tone (see **Table 1**).

Glutamate

Glutamate signaling also plays an important role in sleep, in particular, during the thalamocortical slow oscillations of non-REM (NREM) sleep. Glutamate deficiency is also linked to depression. It is argued that glutamate has a neuroprotective role that is mediated via brain-derived neural growth factor and that low levels of glutamate lead to cell death in areas of the brain responsible for mood regulation. Some antidepressant medications, in particular, selective serotonin reuptake inhibitors such as fluoxetine, have a positive allosteric effect on α-amino-3-hydroxy-5-methyl-4-isoxazolepropionic acid receptor subtype of glutamate receptor.[7]

Hypothalamic-pituitary-adrenal Axis

Proper functioning of the hypothalamic-pituitary-adrenal axis is required for appropriate sleep regulation.[13] Cortisol secretion is decreased during normal deep sleep, and administration of corticotrophin-releasing hormone produces increased arousals and poor sleep particularly in middle-age or older patients. Cortisol replacement is necessary for cortisol-deficient patients to have normal REM sleep. However, direct cortisol administration to non–cortisol-deficient patients seems to decrease REM sleep and increase slow wave sleep (SWS). Some evidence suggests that patients with primary insomnia have elevated levels of cortisol. Hypercortisolemia is also commonly observed in patients with depression. Treatment with selective-serotonin reuptake inhibitors is found to normalize salivary cortisol in depressed patients with hypercortisolemia, although the decrease in cortisol is only weakly associated with improvement in depressive symptoms.[14]

SLEEP DISTURBANCES IN MAJOR DEPRESSIVE DISORDER

A large and occasionally contradictory body of literature describes sleep findings associated with major depressive disorder. The most common subjective sleep complaints elicited from patients with major depressive disorder are insomnia (up to 88%) and hypersomnia (27%).[15] Insomnia, in particular terminal insomnia, is classically associated with major depressive disorder. The relationship between insomnia and mood symptoms is bidirectional in that poor sleep can precede an episode of major depressive disorder, and depressed mood can disrupt normal sleep patterns.[7] Furthermore, it is 3 times more likely that major depressive disorder will develop in individuals with insomnia than those without.[16] In addition, hypersomnia, fatigue, and sleepiness are closely correlated with depressive symptomology.[15] Complaints of nonrestorative sleep and excessive daytime sleepiness can be elicited from many subjects; however, these findings are not universal.[7] In addition, many patients with major depressive disorder have poor insight into their sleep quality, often misestimating their sleep latency, sleep time, and sleep duration.[17]

POLYSOMNOGRAPHY
Polysomnographic Findings in Major Depressive Disorder

Polysomnographic studies have found that major depressive disorder is associated with abnormal sleep architecture. Patients may have prolonged sleep onset latency and frequent nocturnal awakenings resulting in sleep fragmentation and poor sleep efficiency.[7] Depressed patients often have decreased REM sleep latency and prolonged REM sleep periods early in the night, leading to an overall increase in the proportion of REM sleep.[18] In addition, REM sleep in depressed patients is characterized by more frequent rapid eye movements than REM sleep in control patients.[7] The increased number of rapid eye movements normalizes when patients go into remission, whereas the decreased REM sleep latency persists.[19] In addition, decreased REM sleep latency has also been noted in unaffected first-degree relatives. This finding suggests a possible genetic link between REM sleep latency and major depressive disorder. The relative excess of REM sleep seems to come at the expense of stage N3 sleep, also known as slow wave sleep. Not only is time spent in SWS decreased in depressed patients compared with controls, but the distribution of slow wave activity (SWA), a marker of SWS intensity, is abnormal. Control subjects have maximal SWA during the first sleep cycle, whereas depressed patients have peak SWA during subsequent cycles.[20] Unlike REM sleep findings, SWS findings in major depressive disorder are age dependent in that they often cannot be reliably found until patients reach the fifth decade of life.[20] Some research suggests that these findings may be linked to specific subtypes of major depressive disorder. In particular, decreased SWA in the first sleep cycle is more commonly seen in atypical depression than melancholic depression.[7] Although further research is needed, polysomnography may eventually be useful in guiding the choice of pharmacologic agent in depressed patients.

Polysomnography and Primary Sleep Disorders

Polysomnography is not routinely used in the evaluation of depressed or insomniac patients. However, polysomnography may be indicated in patients for whom there is a strong suspicion for a primary sleep disorder. Obstructive sleep apnea (OSA) can produce many of the symptoms of major depressive disorder, including fatigue, depressed mood, and difficulty concentrating.[21] In patients with depression, comorbid sleep apnea can aggravate mood symptoms and make them refractory to treatment. This is particularly relevant because patients with major depressive disorder may be at increased risk for OSA and vice versa.[21] Many patients experience weight gain while taking psychotropic medication, and increased body mass is correlated with increased rates of OSA. In patients with depression and OSA, sedating antidepressants, hypnotics, and benzodiazepines should be used sparingly or avoided entirely, because these drugs can worsen apneic symptoms. Polysomnography may also be considered in depressed patients who present with evidence of a new or worsened restless legs syndrome, periodic limb movement, or REM sleep behavior

disorder, as antidepressant medication can induce or exacerbate these conditions.[22]

PHARMACOLOGIC STRATEGIES

Several studies have found better outcomes when major depressive disorder and associated sleep complaints are addressed in concert. Depressed patients with concomitant sleep disturbances are more likely to have suicidal ideation and more severe symptoms and be refractory to treatment.[7] Furthermore, even in individuals who do respond to antidepressant therapy, persistent insomnia in the absence of current mood symptoms is a strong predictor of future relapse.[23] This is especially concerning given that insomnia is among the most commonly reported residual symptoms during remission for major depressive disorder.[23] Similarly, residual hypersomnia is also commonly encountered and is also associated with an increased risk of relapse.[8]

Hypnotics and Sedating Agents

Insomnia is a common problem, even in individuals who do not have major depressive disorder, and many techniques have been used to address it. Behavioral techniques, such as improving sleep hygiene (see later discussion), are typically the first-line treatments, but several different medications are frequently used as adjuncts. Although benzodiazepines have classically been used to treat insomnia, newer nonbenzodiazepine γ-aminobutyric acid agonists receptor potentiating agents such as zaleplon, zolpidem, and eszopiclone are increasingly popular.[24] Melatonin and melatonin-agonists (ramelteon) are also used and may be especially useful in patients for whom excess sedation is a concern. Many people with insomnia are prescribed sedating antidepressants, typically in doses that are much smaller than when used for mood symptoms. The tricyclic antidepressants, amitriptyline and doxepin, the tetracyclic antidepressant, mirtazapine, and the serotonin antagonist and reuptake inhibitor, trazodone, are the most commonly used drugs in this context.[24] Despite their widespread use, the appropriateness of using antidepressant medications to treat insomnia in nondepressed individuals remains controversial.[25] In contrast to patients with a primary sleep complaint of insomnia, patients complaining of isolated hypersomnia have been treated with stimulants or with modafinil.[7]

Antidepressant Therapy

Pharmacologic management of coincident depression and sleep complaints can be challenging. Most antidepressant medications have some effect on sleep regulation, either sedating or activating (see **Table 1**); therefore, effective treatment of mood symptoms may aggravate existing sleep disturbances or provoke new sleep problems. The situation is further complicated by the observation that each individual responds uniquely to a given medication; therefore, drugs that are typically activating can actually be sedating and vice versa.[7] As a first-line therapy, most clinicians try to determine the optimal dosing of a single agent to address both mood and sleep complaints. This dosing enhances adherence and eliminates the possibility of drug-drug interactions. In addition to their sedating quality, tricyclic antidepressants reverse many of the REM sleep changes observed in depressed patients.[26] However, because of the risk of intentional overdose, tricyclic antidepressants must be used cautiously in patients who have severe depression. Monoamine oxidase inhibitors (MAOIs) such as selegiline can suppress REM sleep. However, it is unclear whether the decreased REM sleep seen with MAOIs or tricyclics is associated with their effects on mood. Selective serotonin reuptake inhibitors, although effective in treating mood symptoms, are more likely to aggravate the polysomnographic abnormalities in depressed sleep and are unlikely to provide lasting sleep benefits.[26] Furthermore, selective serotonin reuptake inhibitors are frequently reported to cause insomnia.[7] Trazodone and mirtazapine are been successfully used as monotherapies to treat insomnia and depression in some patients.[27] Some investigators advocate that patients who have insomnia while taking selective serotonin reuptake inhibitors, bupropion, or venlafaxine should be switched to a sedating antidepressant like trazodone.[27]

Combination Therapy

Many patients have symptoms that cannot be adequately controlled by a single agent. For these patients, adjunct measures must be used. Psychotherapy has been used to treat insomnia accompanied by major depressive disorder. Combining escitalopram with cognitive-behavioral therapy specifically geared toward treating insomnia (see later discussion) provided greater remission from both sleep and mood symptoms than escitalopram alone.[11] Additional antidepressant medication is sometimes used to manage sleep complaints that are resistant or secondary to treatment. The most common such scenario is when low-dose trazodone is added to patients who have insomnia secondary to use of a selective serotonin reuptake

inhibitor.[27] Mirtazapine is also frequently used for this purpose. If the addition of a sedating antidepressant is inappropriate for a given patient, zaleplon, zolpidem, or eszopiclone may be used. A recent randomized, controlled trial found that the addition of eszopiclone to fluoxetine produced statistically significant improvements in subjective sleep quality and wakefulness after sleep onset, total sleep time, and sleep efficiency.[28] Finally, benzodiazepines may be used. However, these agents may be addictive and development of tolerance is also a concern.

NONPHARMACOLOGIC STRATEGIES
Psychotherapy and Sleep Hygiene for Insomnia

Cognitive behavioral therapy for insomnia (CBTI) can be a useful adjunct or alternative to pharmacologic therapy in patients with primary insomnia.[11,29] CBTI has several components, each of which plays a role in improving sleep. One component is stimulus control techniques, which are used to strengthen the connection between the bed and sleep. These include only using the bed for sleep and sex, only getting into bed when tired, leaving the bed if unable to fall asleep within 15 minutes, establishing a regular morning waking time, and avoiding napping.[30] CBTI can also include restrictions on the amount of time in bed.[30] In this case, baseline polysomnography or a sleep diary can be used to assess total sleep time. Initially, the patient is restricted to spending an amount of time in bed equal to their baseline total sleep time. Regular sleep studies or sleep diaries can be used to assess sleep efficiency. If sleep efficiency is greater than 85%, then the amount of time in bed is lengthened by 15 minutes, otherwise the amount of time in bed is decreased by 15 minutes. However, time in bed should be maintained at greater than 5 hours regardless of sleep efficiency. Cognitive therapies such as distraction techniques and cognitive restructuring can address negative and counterproductive beliefs about sleep.[30] Paradoxic intention, in which patients who fear insomnia intentionally stay awake, may be effective for some patients by reducing worry about the negative outcomes from an instance of poor sleep.[30] Several different relaxation therapies may also be used to address insomnia, although these are reported to be less effective than the other CBT techniques described above.[30] In progressive muscle relaxation, patients tense and then relax muscles, concentrating on the way the muscle relaxation feels. Patients may also be taught to breathe with their abdomen (diaphragmatic breathing) while in bed. This pattern of breathing is soothing and occurs naturally during sleep onset. Biofeedback techniques and guided imagery may also help some patients.[30] CBTI and stimulus control techniques and cognitive therapies are found to have an efficacy comparable to or greater than standard pharmacotherapy for insomnia.

Psychotherapy for Insomnia and Depression

Given its success in treating insomnia, researchers have attempted to use CBTI in patients with depression and concomitant insomnia. In a small study, patients with mild depression (Beck Depression Index >9) and insomnia received 6 weekly sessions of CBTI consisting of sleep hygiene education, stimulus control techniques, and progressive muscle relaxation. At a 3-month follow-up visit, all of the patients who had completed CBTI were no longer experiencing clinically significant insomnia and 7 of 8 subjects were no longer in a depressive episode.[29] These benefits were preserved at a 3-month follow-up. A subsequent randomized, controlled trial found that CBTI had an additive effect when combined with escitalopram in the treatment of depression with insomnia.[11] Furthermore, this study found that the combination of escitalopram and CBTI was superior to the combination of escitalopram and a control therapy consisting of sleep hygiene education and a quasi-desensitization procedure for treating both depressed mood and insomnia.

Sleep Deprivation and Major Depressive Disorder

Several studies found positive effects of sleep deprivation on depression symptoms. Multiple studies have shown that a single night of total sleep deprivation (TSD) produces positive results in up to 50% of subjects.[31] This response rate is comparable to what can be achieved with antidepressant medications. Furthermore, TSD responders show benefits comparable with those observed with pharmacotherapy.[31] Patients with melancholic depression, characterized by terminal insomnia and diurnal variation of symptoms, are more likely to respond to TSD than patients with atypical or seasonal depression.[7] Imaging studies suggest that TSD responders have increased metabolism in the amygdala, orbital prefrontal gyrus, and inferior temporal and anterior cingulate cortices, which normalizes after sleep deprivation.[31] Intriguingly, the degree of hypermetabolism in these regions is correlated to the response to TSD. However, response to TSD is unpredictable in that prior positive responses do not predict future responses.[32] Furthermore, even in patients for whom it is

effective, TSD is not a practical therapeutic intervention because the benefits dissipate after recovery sleep.[32] This has led researchers to study more sustainable ways of scheduling sleep to improve depression.

Partial sleep deprivation (PSD), including deprivation of REM sleep, deprivation of SWS, and disruption of individual slow waves have all demonstrated mild-to-moderate improvements in depression scores.[31,33] Because of the interrelated nature of these sleep parameters, it is difficult to say how much of the observed antidepressant effects in these studies are directly mediated by the parameters that were manipulated or which component of TSD is necessary. Additionally, the effects of PSD are not necessarily the same as the improvements after acute TSD.[31] In particular, several weeks of PSD produces a gradual improvement in mood symptoms, which persists longer than TSD although will eventually diminish when the therapy is discontinued.[34] Circadian phase shifting is found to improve depression symptoms.[35] Other studies have found benefits for combination therapies. Combining TSD with circadian rhythm interventions or light therapy can prolong the antidepressant effects of TSD. Both PSD and TSD potentiate the effects of selective serotonin reuptake inhibitors and tricyclics.[31] Although sleep scheduling techniques are promising avenues of research, they remain experimental and are not yet part of standard medical practice.

REFERENCES

1. Blazer DG, Kessler RC, McGonagle KA, et al. The prevalence and distribution of major depression in a national community sample: the national comorbidity survey. Am J Psychiatry 1994;151(7): 979–86.

2. Krishnan KR, Delong M, Kraemer H, et al. Comorbidity of depression with other medical diseases in the elderly. Biol Psychiatry 2002;52(6):559–88.

3. McIntyre RS, O'Donovan C. The human cost of not achieving full remission in depression. Can J Psychiatry 2004;49(1):10–6.

4. Stewart WF, Ricci JA, Chee E, et al. Cost of lost productive work time among US workers with depression. JAMA 2003;289(23):3135–44.

5. Rush AJ, Trivedi MH, Wisniewski SR, et al. Acute and longer-term outcomes in depressed outpatients requiring one or several treatment steps: a STAR* D report. Am J Psychiatry 2006;163(11):1905–17.

6. American Psychiatric Association. Task Force on DSM-IV. Diagnostic and statistical manual of mental disorders: DSM-IV-TR. Arlington, VA: American Psychiatric Publishing, Inc; 2000.

7. Peterson MJ, Benca RM. Sleep in mood disorders. Sleep Med Clin 2008;3(2):231–49.

8. Kaplan KA, Harvey AG. Hypersomnia across mood disorders: a review and synthesis. Sleep Med Rev 2009;13(4):275–85.

9. Baglioni C, Battagliese G, Feige B, et al. Insomnia as a predictor of depression: a meta-analytic evaluation of longitudinal epidemiological studies. J Affect Disord 2011;135:10–9.

10. McCall WV, Blocker JN, D'Agostino R Jr, et al. Treatment of insomnia in depressed insomniacs: effects on health-related quality of life, objective and self-reported sleep, and depression. J Clin Sleep Med 2010;6(4):322–9.

11. Manber R, Edinger JD, Gress JL, et al. Cognitive behavioral therapy for insomnia enhances depression outcome in patients with comorbid major depressive disorder and insomnia. Sleep 2008; 31(4):489–95.

12. Pace-Schott EF, Hobson JA. The neurobiology of sleep: genetics, cellular physiology and subcortical networks. Nat Rev Neurosci 2002;3(8):591–605.

13. Vgontzas AN, Chrousos GP. Sleep, the hypothalamic-pituitary-adrenal axis, and cytokines: multiple interactions and disturbances in sleep disorders. Endocrinol Metab Clin North Am 2002;31(1):15–36.

14. Hinkelmann K, Moritz S, Botzenhardt J, et al. Changes in cortisol secretion during antidepressive treatment and cognitive improvement in patients with major depression: a longitudinal study. Psychoneuroendocrinology 2012;37(5):685–92.

15. Yates WR, Mitchell J, Rush AJ, et al. Clinical features of depressed outpatients with and without co-occurring general medical conditions in STAR* D. Gen Hosp Psychiatry 2004;26(6):421–9.

16. Johnson EO, Roth T, Breslau N. The association of insomnia with anxiety disorders and depression: exploration of the direction of risk. J Psychiatr Res 2006;40(8):700–8.

17. Matousek M, Cervena K, Zavesicka L, et al. Subjective and objective evaluation of alertness and sleep quality in depressed patients. BMC Psychiatry 2004;4(1):14.

18. Benca RM, Obermeyer WH, Thisted RA, et al. Sleep and psychiatric disorders: a meta-analysis. Arch Gen Psychiatry 1992;49(8):651–68.

19. Thase ME, Fasiczka AL, Berman SR, et al. Electroencephalographic sleep profiles before and after cognitive behavior therapy of depression. Arch Gen Psychiatry 1998;55:138–44.

20. Kupfer DJ, Frank E, Mc Eachran A, et al. Delta sleep ratio. Arch Gen Psychiatry 1990;47:1100–5.

21. Schröder C, O'Hara R. Depression and obstructive sleep apnea (OSA). Ann Gen Psychiatry 2005;4:13.

22. Sculthorpe LD, Douglass AB. Sleep pathologies in depression and the clinical utility of polysomnography. Can J Psychiatry 2010;55(7):413–21.

23. Benca RM, Peterson MJ. Insomnia and depression. Sleep Med 2008;9:S3–9.

24. Schutte-Rodin S, Broch L, Buysse D, et al. Clinical guideline for the evaluation and management of chronic insomnia in adults. J Clin Sleep Med 2008; 4(5):487–504.

25. Wiegand MH. Antidepressants for the treatment of insomnia: a suitable approach? Drugs 2008;68(17): 2411–7.

26. Argyropoulos SV, Wilson SJ. Sleep disturbances in depression and the effects of antidepressants. Int Rev Psychiatry 2005;17(4):237–45.

27. Jindal RD, Thase ME. Treatment of insomnia associated with clinical depression. Sleep Med Rev 2004; 8(1):19–30.

28. Fava M, McCall WV, Krystal A, et al. Eszopiclone co-administered with fluoxetine in patients with insomnia coexisting with major depressive disorder. Biol Psychiatry 2006;59(11):1052–60.

29. Taylor DJ, Lichstein KL, Weinstock J, et al. A pilot study of cognitive-behavioral therapy of insomnia in people with mild depression. Behav Ther 2007; 38(1):49–57.

30. Perlis ML, Smith MT, Jungquist C, et al. Cognitive behavioral therapy for insomnia. In: Attarian HP, Schuman S, editors. Clin Handbook Insomnia. Second Edition. New York, NY: Humana Press; 2010. p. 281–96.

31. Benedetti F, Columbo C. Sleep deprivation in mood disorders. Neuropsychobiology 2011;64(3):141–51.

32. Wirz-Justice A, Van den Hoofdakker RH. Sleep deprivation in depression: what do we know, where do we go? Biol Psychiatry 1999;46(4):445–53.

33. Landsness EC, Goldstein MR, Peterson MJ, et al. Antidepressant effects of selective slow wave sleep deprivation in major depression: a high-density EEG investigation. J Psychiatr Res 2011;45(8):1019–26.

34. Giedke H, Schwärzler F. Therapeutic use of sleep deprivation in depression. Sleep Med Rev 2002; 6(5):361–77.

35. Wirz-Justice A, Benedetti F, Berger M, et al. Chronotherapeutics (light and wake therapy) in affective disorders. Psychol Med 2005;35(7):939–44.

Sleep and Mood During Pregnancy and the Postpartum Period

Bei Bei, DPsych, PhD[a,b], Soledad Coo, PhD[a],
John Trinder, PhD[a,*]

KEYWORDS

• Pregnancy • Postpartum • Perinatal • Mood • Sleep • Depression • Anxiety

KEY POINTS

- Based on self-report and objective assessments, sleep is disrupted during pregnancy and the postpartum period.
- There is strong evidence that poor self-reported sleep quality is associated with poor mood and might be a risk factor for mood problems during the perinatal period.
- The relationship between objectively assessed sleep and mood is weaker and less consistent than the relationship between subjective sleep and mood.
- Nonpharmacologic intervention studies have shown promise in improving maternal sleep and mood.

PERINATAL MOOD DISTURBANCES

Despite commonly held beliefs of joy and happiness, women are vulnerable to mood disturbances during the perinatal period. Postpartum blues, or baby blues, is a transient form of moodiness experienced by up to 85% of new mothers 3 to 4 days after delivery, which usually dissipates within a week.[1] A smaller but notable percentage of new mothers experience a major depressive disorder during pregnancy (up to 20%) or the postpartum period (about 12%–16%).[2] Although postpartum blues is generally considered a normal event that does not impair functioning, perinatal depression is a psychiatric condition that requires clinical attention.

The exact causes of postpartum blues and perinatal depression are under ongoing research. Serum levels of many circulating hormones (eg, estrogen, progesterone, prolactin, thyroid hormones) increase gradually over the course of pregnancy and then decrease precipitously within days of delivery,[3] followed by a slower retreat from extravascular compartments.[4] These changes coincide with the occurrence of perinatal mood disturbances, but neither single nor combined biochemical factors have been identified as direct contributors. Several psychosocial factors have been shown to increase the risk for perinatal mood disturbances, including antenatal anxiety and depressive symptoms, the presence of psychiatric history, marital conflict, lack of social support, and stressful life events.[5]

Sleep disturbance has only recently been studied as a possible contributing factor to perinatal mood disturbances. This article describes the effect of the perinatal period on the sleep of mothers and reviews the literature relating disrupted sleep and perinatal mood disturbances.

SLEEP DURING PREGNANCY AND THE POSTPARTUM PERIOD
Methods of Sleep Measurement

In this literature, sleep has been assessed by a variety of methods, each with advantages and disadvantages. Subjective measurements of sleep

[a] Melbourne School of Psychological Sciences, University of Melbourne, Gratton Street, Parkville, Victoria 3010, Australia; [b] School of Psychological Sciences, Monash University, Mount Waverley, Victoria 3149, Australia
* Corresponding author.
E-mail address: johnat@unimelb.edu.au

Sleep Med Clin 10 (2015) 25–33
http://dx.doi.org/10.1016/j.jsmc.2014.11.011
1556-407X/15/$ – see front matter © 2015 Elsevier Inc. All rights reserved.

include self-report questionnaires, rating scales, and sleep diaries and are the most widely used methods in childbearing women. Subjective methods are nonintrusive and easy to administer. They reflect women's overall perception rather than an accurate assessment of actual sleep.

Objective sleep assessment typically involves polysomnography (PSG) and/or actigraphy. PSG is an electrophysiological study of sleep that collects physiologic information and plots them against time. Although typically conducted in a sleep laboratory, in a perinatal population, PSG is more commonly used in an ambulatory form in a woman's own home. Although PSG gives detailed assessments of sleep duration and quality, as well as sleep architecture, it is compromised by a relatively higher cost as well as involving an unnatural sleeping environment as a result of equipment discomfort. An actigraph is a watchlike device that estimates sleep duration and quality based on wrist movement. It is capable of continuous measurement of sleep over multiple days or even weeks in participants' natural environment with minimum intrusion.

Studies have shown differences between self-report, PSG, and actigraphy-measured sleep parameters. For example, self-reported sleep duration has been found to be longer than that measured by actigraphy[6] and PSG[7] during the second and third trimesters, whereas self-reported sleep-onset latency (SOL) was found to be longer than that measured by PSG in both pregnant and nonpregnant women.[7]

Sleep Characteristics During the Perinatal Period

Sleep and wake patterns are significantly challenged during the perinatal period. New mothers are exposed to possible chronic sleep disruption and fragmentation during pregnancy, acute sleep deprivation during labor and immediate postpartum periods, as well as chronic partial sleep deprivation and disruption during the first few months after giving birth to the newborn.

Subjective sleep

In cross-sectional studies, pregnant women have self-reported poorer sleep than nonpregnant controls.[8] Longitudinal studies provide insight into specific changes in sleep over the perinatal period. For example, in a study of 325 pregnant women with sleep measured by self-report, there was an increase in nighttime awakenings and a decrease in sleep efficiency (SE) beginning in the first trimester and continuing throughout pregnancy. Perceived total sleep time (TST) increased during the first trimester and then slightly decreased during the second trimester, followed by a substantial decrease during late pregnancy.[9] This finding suggests that women perceive their sleep to be disrupted from as early as the first trimester despite an increase in sleep duration. Sleep tends to gradually improve during the postpartum period. In a small study ($N = 7$), sleep diaries kept continuously from 5 to 12 weeks post partum showed a progressive decrease in wake after sleep onset.[10] The same study also noted that from 9 to 12 weeks post partum, women's sleep patterns were associated with their reports of infant sleep-wake patterns and feeding practices.

Objective sleep

Cross-sectional PSG studies have revealed significant differences in sleep architecture in pregnant women compared with nonpregnant controls. One of the earliest studies[11] compared PSG measures of 7 women in the last month of pregnancy with 9 age-matched nonpregnant controls and found that the pregnant group had longer SOL, more nighttime awakenings, less TST, and less slow wave sleep (SWS). A similar study[12] compared 12 women in the third trimester to 10 nonpregnant controls and found that pregnant women had lower SE largely caused by nighttime awakenings, more stage 1 sleep, and a lower percentage of rapid-eye-movement (REM) sleep; however, no group differences in TST or SWS were found. Longitudinal PSG studies are rare. Lee and colleagues[13] obtained ambulatory PSG-measured sleep in 31 women before pregnancy, at each trimester, and at 1 and 3 months post partum. The TST was the lowest at 1 month post partum, averaging 6.2 hours, followed by the third trimester and prepregnancy baseline, and was the highest during the first trimester, averaging 7.4 hours. SE decreased progressively across pregnancy, from 93% before pregnancy to 81% at 1 month post partum. There was no significant difference in REM sleep over time, but SWS progressively decreased throughout pregnancy. A general improving trend in all aspects of sleep was observed at 3 months post partum, although neither sleep quality nor quantity returned to prepregnancy levels.

Studies using actigraphy have confirmed the PSG finding that nighttime sleep deteriorates progressively throughout pregnancy, particularly during the last weeks of gestation, being the poorest on the night before delivery.[14,15] A recent actigraphy study[16] of the weeks immediately before and after delivery reported that, although nighttime sleep was significantly disrupted after giving birth, napping significantly increased, resulting in the

TST across 24 hours remaining relatively stable (**Fig. 1**). Unlike the antenatal period, when naps were most likely to occur during early afternoon, during the first postpartum week, naps were evenly distributed across late morning to early evening (**Fig. 2**). These findings suggest that immediately after giving birth, sleep was redistributed across 24-hour periods, raising questions as to the restorative value of sleep new mothers obtain. Similar to findings in PSG studies, actigraphy-measured sleep showed an improving trend further into the postpartum period, with reports that at 10 weeks post partum, sleep patterns were similar to that in the third trimester, although sleep quality was still worse than matched controls.[14]

Factors that Affect Sleep During the Perinatal Period

Several factors contribute to the changes in sleep during the perinatal periods described earlier (see Lee[17] for an earlier review).

Physiologic alterations

Elevated levels of progesterone during pregnancy have been associated with increased daytime sleepiness and shorter SOL during the first trimester. Some have also suggested that progesterone might have an inhibitory effect on smooth muscles, leading to increased urinary frequency during early pregnancy.[17] Physical discomforts during pregnancy have been widely acknowledged as sleep disrupting.[18] These discomforts include increased urination, nausea, tender breasts, headache, vaginal discharge, flatulence, constipation, shortness of breath, backache, and heartburn.[17] These symptoms often persist throughout pregnancy with varying degrees of severity and can lead to sleep disruption.

Sleep disorders

Increased prevalence of some sleep disorders during pregnancy has been linked to sleep fragmentation and increased daytime sleepiness among affected women. A study of 502 pregnancies[19] reported regular snoring in 23% of the sample, whereas only 4% of the same sample reported regular snoring before pregnancy. Changes in the respiratory system during pregnancy, such as reduced pharyngeal dimensions,[20] decreased nasal patency, and increased congestion and rhinitis,[21] have been proposed as potential contributors to snoring. The prevalence of restless legs syndrome (RLS) has been observed to increase during pregnancy[22] and to resolve rapidly post partum.[23] A large cross-sectional study involving approximately 16,000 pregnant women[24] found that 15% reported RLS symptoms at 3 to 4 months of gestation, which increased to 23% at term. Iron deficiency and serum folate levels have been investigated as contributing factors.[22]

Infant behavior

The various needs of the newborn are the main contributing factors to sleep disruptions during the postpartum period. Feeding and caretaking often lead to multiple nighttime awakenings in new parents and more so when temperament of the infant is difficult.[25,26] Actigraphy studies have shown that maternal sleep was closely associated with infant sleep/wake behaviors during the first 3 months post partum.[10,27] In addition, the number of self-report infant-related nighttime awakenings, but not the self-estimated total wake time, was found to be associated with perceived sleep quality,[28] highlighting the role of sleep disruption over reduced TST in perceived sleep quality.

Labor

As would be anticipated, birth-giving, especially nighttime labor, has been associated with acute sleep deprivation throughout delivery and the week immediately afterward. Some studies have reported that caesarean sections were associated with shorter TST and more frequent nighttime awakenings than vaginal deliveries, probably because of discomfort and other factors related to surgical recovery.[29]

Parity

Parity has not been shown to have a consistent effect on sleep. Some investigators have described multiparas mothers as having less efficient sleep than nulliparas from before pregnancy until 3 months post partum, mainly because of an increased number of brief nocturnal awakenings,[30] whereas others[31] have observed a greater deterioration in objective sleep and increased number of daytime naps in nulliparas during the third trimester and 1 week post partum. Although no differences have been reported in objective TST, percentage of REM sleep, and percentage of SWS, multiparas tend to initiate SWS quicker than nulliparas.[13]

SLEEP AND PERINATAL MOOD DISTURBANCES

Changes in sleep during the perinatal period coincide with the occurrence of perinatal mood disturbances. Given the intimate relationship between sleep disturbances and mood in the nonpregnant population,[32] several studies have assessed the impact of sleep on mood among new mothers.

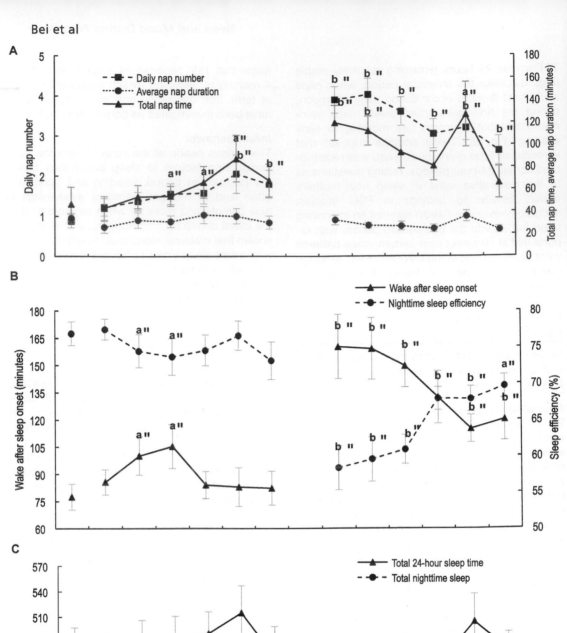

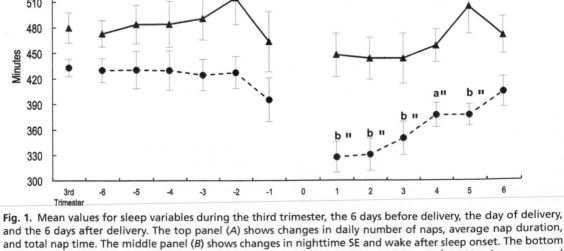

Fig. 1. Mean values for sleep variables during the third trimester, the 6 days before delivery, and the day of delivery, and the 6 days after delivery. The top panel (*A*) shows changes in daily number of naps, average nap duration, and total nap time. The middle panel (*B*) shows changes in nighttime SE and wake after sleep onset. The bottom panel (*C*) shows changes in total nighttime sleep and total 24-hour sleep. N = 24, [a] $P<.05$, [b] $P<.01$, when compared with the third-trimester value using paired sample t tests. (*Data from* Coo Calcagni S, Bei B, Milgrom J, et al. The relationship between sleep and mood in first-time and experienced mothers. Behav Sleep Med 2012;10:167–79.)

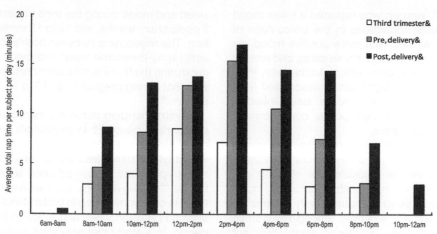

Fig. 2. Time spent napping as a function of perinatal phase (third trimester, predelivery, and postdelivery) and time of day (2-hour intervals between 6 AM and 12 AM). Calculated as average time spent napping per subject and per day for each of the 2-hour intervals. N = 24. (*Data from* Coo Calcagni S, Bei B, Milgrom J, et al. The relationship between sleep and mood in first-time and experienced mothers. Behav Sleep Med 2012;10:167–79.)

Sleep Measured Subjectively

Most studies that have explored the relationship between sleep and mood during the perinatal period measured sleep subjectively and found poor perceived sleep quality to be more common among women with higher levels of depressive symptoms than nondepressed women during pregnancy.[33] A study comparing clinically depressed and nondepressed pregnant women[34] found that, although fragmented sleep was more frequently reported by depressed women during mid to late pregnancy overall, both depressed and nondepressed women reported their sleep to be disturbed at 36 weeks' gestation This finding suggests that, although depression is associated with poorer reported sleep, sleep disturbance is likely a common experience in late pregnancy. With regard to the postpartum period, a study[27] that followed up 124 women from the third trimester to 1, 2, and 3 months post partum found a significant association between reported sleep disruption and depressed mood during the postpartum period. More specifically, postpartum women with higher levels of depressive symptoms reported higher levels of sleep disturbance, reduced TST, increased SOL, more early morning awakenings, and increased daytime sleepiness compared with those with lower depressive symptoms. A similar longitudinal study[35] followed up 38 women from the last trimester to the first year post partum and found that self-reported sleep characteristics during the third trimester, such as increased TST, later rise times, and longer naps, were associated with more depressive symptoms at about 2 to 4 weeks post partum. These results

were inconsistent with previous findings that less TST was associated with poorer mood and suggest a complex interaction between sleep and mood during pregnancy and postpartum periods.

The significant association between sleep complaints and poorer mood during the perinatal period have led to investigations into poor sleep being a risk factor for perinatal depression. A study on 273 pregnant women across the 3 trimesters of pregnancy found that poor subjective sleep quality in the first and second trimesters significantly predicted depressive symptoms in the second and third trimesters, respectively.[36] In 51 women with a history of depression, self-reported poor sleep at 36 weeks' gestation predicted the development of postpartum depression by 4 weeks after childbirth.[37] In addition, sleep complaints across the first 17 postpartum weeks have been associated with a higher risk for recurrent depression in women with prior depressive disorder but who were not depressed during pregnancy.[38] These findings suggest that sleep complaints are not only relevant to concurrent mood during the perinatal periods but might also be a risk factor for future mood problems, particularly among women who are vulnerable to depression.

Sleep Measured Objectively

Few studies have explored the relationship between perinatal mood and sleep using PSG. Lee and colleagues[13] studied the relationship between sleep and depressive symptoms in 31 women who were assessed on 5 occasions: at every trimester of pregnancy and at 3 to 4 and 11 to 12 weeks post partum. From the third trimester to 1 month post partum, women who reported a lower mood showed greater reductions in the percentage of REM sleep; women with more positive mood, on the other hand, had more stable sleep, and smaller increases in percentage wake. Additionally, PSG sleep quality was significantly associated with cognitive functioning, with poorer sleep linked to higher levels of confusion, poorer concentration, and more forgetfulness.

Several recent studies on sleep and mood during the perinatal period incorporated actigraphy as an objective measurement of sleep and reported stronger relationship between mood and self-report sleep compared with actigraphy-assessed sleep. For example, among 160 women in early gestation, a sleep diary, but not actigraphy-assessed sleep deficiency, was found to be significantly associated with more depressive symptoms.[39] A cross-sectional study compared self-report and actigraphy-measured sleep at 3 months post partum among 21 depressed and 21 age- and parity-matched nondepressed mothers.[40] The investigators reported that, although the depressed group reported significantly more sleep complaints compared with the nondepressed group, actigraphy-assessed sleep quality was compromised in both groups and did not differ significantly between the two groups.

It has been noted that although overall the relationship between actigraphy-assessed sleep and mood is weak, it is not the case for all sleep parameters. A recent longitudinal study of 25 healthy nulliparas measured sleep during the third trimester and at the 2nd, 6th, 10th, and 14th postpartum week.[41] Consistent with previous findings, the investigators reported a strong association between self-report sleep and depressive symptoms; the study also reported that, although little relationship was found between actigraphy-measured nighttime sleep duration and depressive symptoms, sleep maintenance parameters measured by actigraphy, such as higher sleep fragmentation and wake after sleep onset (WASO), and lower SE were also significantly correlated with higher depressive symptoms. Tsai and Thomas[42] explored the role of sleep regularity in maternal mood among 26 healthy nulliparas and found that higher variability of actigraphy-assessed nighttime sleep duration was associated with a greater number of symptoms of depression in the first 3 postpartum months. In addition to the type of sleep parameters under question, Coo and colleagues[43] suggested that the strength of the relationship between sleep and mood might vary depending on the timing of assessment. They studied 29 healthy mothers and assessed sleep and mood during the third trimester, the first 2 postpartum weeks, and 10 to 12 weeks post partum. The relationship between both subjective and actigraphy-measured sleep and mood was stronger during the first 2 weeks post partum compared with that during pregnancy or 10 to 12 weeks post partum.[43]

Daytime napping behaviors increase during the postpartum period[16]; in individuals experiencing poor sleep, napping is commonly associated with daytime sleepiness and a conscious effort to make up for the perceived poor sleep the night before.[44] However, few studies have integrated the role of daytime sleep in understanding the relationship between sleep and mood in the perinatal period. In a study that assessed sleep and mood in 44 healthy women from the third trimester to 1 week post partum, Bei and colleagues[45] found that, although actigraphy-measured nighttime sleep quality or duration were not strongly associated with antepartum or postpartum mood, poorer subjective nighttime sleep, higher sleep-related daytime dysfunction, as well as a greater number of daytime naps were significantly associated with mood disturbances during the third trimester and at 1 week post partum. These studies suggest that, in addition to nighttime sleep duration and quality, the awareness of sleep's impact during waking hours might also be critical in the occurrence of perinatal mood disturbances.

INTERVENTION STUDIES

The increasing recognition of the impact of disrupted sleep on new mothers' mood has encouraged intervention studies aimed to improve sleep during the perinatal period. Most of the intervention studies have targeted infant sleep through the delivery of parenting skills with the intention of improving parental sleep and well-being. For example, a randomized controlled study[26] showed that reducing infant sleep problems through behavioral intervention led to significantly decreased maternal depressive symptoms, an effect that was sustained at 4 months after the intervention.

Limited intervention studies have targeted parental sleep. Lee and Gay[46] applied sleep hygiene and bedroom environment improvements in a randomized controlled trial and showed that sleep improved among parents who were less socioeconomically equipped but not among those who were socioeconomically advantaged. A mindful yoga pilot study of 15 nulliparous women reported reduced nighttime awakenings and improved SE in the second, but not the third, trimester.[47] A behavioral- and education-based randomized controlled pilot study with combined interventions for 30 new mothers and their infants reported that the intervention lengthened the infants' longest sleep period and increased the mothers' TST.[48]

Sleep-improving interventions that selectively target women with perinatal mood and sleep problems are currently under development and have shown promising results. An open pilot trial of cognitive behavioral therapy for insomnia (CBTi) has recently been carried out in women with coexisting postpartum depression and insomnia.[49] In this study, 12 women participated in a 5-week individual treatment program covering psycho-education, behavioral strategies for better sleep, sleep hygiene, relaxation, and changing unhelpful thoughts and beliefs about sleep. Modifications to conventional CBTi were made based on postpartum needs, for example, more flexible sleep schedules to accommodate variable infant sleep, allowing naps of short duration and appropriate timing, skills on managing infant sleep, and incorporating partners' support. Comparing measures taken before and after the intervention, there was significant improvement in symptoms of depression, duration and quality of sleep, and fatigue. Despite being a small open trial, this study suggests that a brief course of CBTi tailored to the postpartum period might improve both sleep and mood in new mothers with insomnia and depression.

As there are little data on whether sleep medications are safe for lactating women, and the use of medication often raises concerns in women during the perinatal periods, effective nonpharmacologic treatment of problematic sleep is of particular relevance for perinatal women. Such interventions are further encouraged by the aforementioned findings that subjective perception of sleep shares a stronger relationship with mood problems than its objective duration or quality. Future intervention studies may benefit from incorporating cognitive components that have the potential to alter women's perspectives on pregnancy-related sleep disturbances and install a positive outlook and increase self-efficacy.

SUMMARY

Studies using both objective and subjective methods have confirmed that sleep is disrupted during pregnancy and postpartum periods, with pregnancy-related physical changes, childbirth, and infant care being the most significant contributing factors. The most consistent findings on pregnancy-related sleep changes are (1) a gradual decrease in TST and SE throughout pregnancy; (2) acute sleep deprivation during labor and the immediate postpartum period; and (3) continued compromise for at least 3 months post partum.

Pregnancy-related sleep disruptions are inevitable in the process of becoming a mother. Further, there is strong evidence that self-report sleep complaints are associated with poor mood during the perinatal period, and poor perceived sleep might be a risk factor for both antepartum and postpartum mood disturbances. Findings regarding the relationship between objectively assessed sleep and mood have been mixed, with some studies reporting weak relationships between the two, and some suggesting certain aspects of objective sleep, such as sleep continuity and regularity being related to mood. The stronger relationship between mood and subjectively compared with objectively measured sleep during the perinatal period highlights the importance of women's perception and conscious awareness of poor sleep in their emotional well-being. Future research is needed to address women's subjective experiences of sleep problems, which are likely more susceptible to guidance and changes than the often inevitable and uncontrollable aspects of sleep disruption itself.

REFERENCES

1. O'Hara MW. Post-partum "blues," depression, and psychosis: a review. J Psychosom Obstet Gynaecol 1987;7:205–27.
2. Leung BM, Kaplan BJ. Perinatal depression: prevalence, risks, and the nutrition link–a review of the literature. J Am Diet Assoc 2009;109:1566–75.
3. Deakin J. Motherhood and mental illness. 2nd edition. London: Butterworth; 1988.
4. Ryan KJ, Tulchinsky D. Maternal-fetal endocrinology. Philadelphia: WB Saunders Co; 1980.
5. Pearlstein T, Howard M, Salisbury A, et al. Post-partum depression. Am J Obstet Gynecol 2009;200:357–64.
6. Herring SJ, Foster GD, Pien GW, et al. Do pregnant women accurately report sleep time? A comparison between self-reported and objective measures of sleep duration in pregnancy among a sample of urban mothers. Sleep Breath 2013;17:1323–7.
7. Wilson DL, Fung A, Walker SP, et al. Subjective reports versus objective measurement of sleep latency and sleep duration in pregnancy. Behav Sleep Med 2013;11:207–21.
8. Ko SH, Chang SC, Chen CH. A comparative study of sleep quality between pregnant and nonpregnant Taiwanese women. J Nurs Scholarsh 2010;42:23–30.
9. Hedman C, Pohjasvaara T, Tolonen U, et al. Effects of pregnancy on mothers' sleep. Sleep Med 2002;3:37–42.

10. Horiuchi S, Nishihara K. Analyses of mothers' sleep logs in postpartum periods. Psychiatry Clin Neurosci 1999;53:137–9.

11. Karacan I. Characteristics of sleep patterns during late pregnancy and the postpartum periods. Am J Obstet Gynecol 1968;101:579–86.

12. Hertz G, Fast A, Feinsilver SH, et al. Sleep in normal late pregnancy. Sleep 1992;15:246–51.

13. Lee KA, McEnany G, Zaffke ME. REM sleep and mood state in childbearing women: sleepy or weepy? Sleep 2000;23:877–85.

14. Matsumoto K, Shinkoda H, Kang MJ, et al. Longitudinal study of mothers' sleep-wake behaviors and circadian time patterns from late pregnancy to postpartum: monitoring of wrist actigraphy and sleep logs. Biol Rhythm Res 2003;34:265–78.

15. Beebe KR, Lee KA. Sleep disturbance in late pregnancy and early labor. J Perinat Neonatal Nurs 2007;21:103–8.

16. Bei B, Coo Calcagni S, Milgrom J, et al. Day-to-day alteration of 24-hour sleep pattern immediately before and after giving birth. Sleep and Biological Rhythms 2012;10:212.

17. Lee KA. Alterations in sleep during pregnancy and postpartum: a review of 30 years of research. Sleep Med Rev 1998;2:231–42.

18. Kamysheva E, Skouteris H, Wertheim EH, et al. A prospective investigation of the relationships among sleep quality, physical symptoms, and depressive symptoms during pregnancy. J Affect Disord 2010;123:317–20.

19. Franklin KA, Holmgren PA, Jönsson F, et al. Snoring, pregnancy-induced hypertension, and growth retardation of the fetus. Chest 2000;117:137–41.

20. Pilkington S, Carli F, Dakin MJ, et al. Increase in Mallampati score during pregnancy. Br J Anaesth 1995; 74:638–42.

21. Bende M, Gredmark T. Nasal stuffiness during pregnancy. Laryngoscope 1999;109:1108–10.

22. Lee KA, Zaffke ME, Baratte-Beebe K. Restless legs syndrome and sleep disturbance during pregnancy: the role of folate and iron. J Womens Health Gend Based Med 2001;10:335–41.

23. Goodman JD, Brodie C, Ayida GA. Restless leg syndrome in pregnancy. BMJ 1988;297:1101–2.

24. Suzuki K, Ohida T, Sone T, et al. The prevalence of restless legs syndrome among pregnant women in Japan and the relationship between restless legs syndrome and sleep problems. Sleep 2003; 26:673–7.

25. Dennis CL, Ross L. Relationships among infant sleep patterns, maternal fatigue, and development of depressive symptomatology. Birth 2005; 32:187–93.

26. Hiscock H, Wake M. Infant sleep problems and postnatal depression: a community-based study. Pediatrics 2001;107:1317–22.

27. Goyal D, Gay CL, Lee KA. Patterns of sleep disruption and depressive symptoms in new mothers. J Perinat Neonatal Nurs 2007;21:123–9.

28. Gress JL, Chambers AS, Ong JC, et al. Maternal subjective sleep quality and nighttime infant care. J Reprod Infant Psychol 2010;28:384–91.

29. Lee SY, Lee KA. Early postpartum sleep and fatigue for mothers after cesarean delivery compared with vaginal delivery: an exploratory study. J Perinat Neonatal Nurs 2007;21:109–13.

30. Lee KA, Zaffke ME, McEnany G. Parity and sleep patterns during and after pregnancy. Obstet Gynecol 2000;95:14–8.

31. Coo Calcagni S, Bei B, Milgrom J, et al. The relationship between sleep and mood in first-time and experienced mothers. Behav Sleep Med 2012;10:167–79.

32. Alvaro PK, Roberts RM, Harris JK. A systematic review assessing bidirectionality between sleep disturbances, anxiety, and depression. Sleep 2013;36: 1059–68.

33. Jomeen J, Martin CR. Assessment and relationship of sleep quality to depression in early pregnancy. J Reprod Infant Psychol 2007;25:87–99.

34. Okun ML, Kiewra K, Luther JF, et al. Sleep disturbances in depressed and nondepressed pregnant women. Depress Anxiety 2011;28:676–85.

35. Wolfson AR, Crowley SJ, Anwer U, et al. Changes in sleep patterns and depressive symptoms in first-time mothers: last trimester to 1-year postpartum. Behav Sleep Med 2003;1:54–67.

36. Skouteris H, Germano C, Wertheim EH, et al. Sleep quality and depression during pregnancy: a prospective study. J Sleep Res 2008;17:217–20.

37. Okun ML, Hanusa BH, Hall M, et al. Sleep complaints in late pregnancy and the recurrence of postpartum depression. Behav Sleep Med 2009;7: 106–17.

38. Okun ML, Luther J, Prather AA, et al. Changes in sleep quality, but not hormones predict time to postpartum depression recurrence. J Affect Disord 2011;130:378–84.

39. Okun ML, Kline CE, Roberts JM, et al. Prevalence of sleep deficiency in early gestation and its associations with stress and depressive symptoms. J Womens Health (Larchmt) 2013;22:1028–37.

40. Dørheim SK, Bondevik GT, Eberhard-Gran M, et al. Subjective and objective sleep among depressed and non-depressed postnatal women. Acta Psychiatr Scand 2009;119:128–36.

41. Park EM, Meltzer-Brody S, Stickgold R. Poor sleep maintenance and subjective sleep quality are associated with postpartum maternal depression symptom severity. Arch Womens Ment Health 2013;16: 539–47.

42. Tsai SY, Thomas KA. Sleep disturbances and depressive symptoms in healthy postpartum women: a pilot study. Res Nurs Health 2012;35:314–23.

43. Coo S, Milgrom J, Trinder J. Mood and objective and subjective measures of sleep during late pregnancy and the postpartum period. Behav Sleep Med 2014; 12:317–30.

44. Harvey AG. A cognitive model of insomnia. Behav Res Ther 2002;40:869–93.

45. Bei B, Milgrom J, Ericksen J, et al. Subjective perception of sleep, but not its objective quality, is associated with immediate postpartum mood disturbances in healthy women. Sleep 2010;33: 531–8.

46. Lee KA, Gay CL. Can modifications to the bedroom environment improve the sleep of new parents? Two randomized controlled trials. Res Nurs Health 2011; 34:7–19.

47. Beddoe AE, Lee KA, Weiss SJ, et al. Effects of mindful yoga on sleep in pregnant women: a pilot study. Biol Res Nurs 2010;11:363–70.

48. Stremler R, Hodnett E, Lee K, et al. A behavioral-educational intervention to promote maternal and infant sleep: a pilot randomized, controlled trial. Sleep 2006;29:1609–15.

49. Swanson LM, Flynn H, Adams-Mundy JD, et al. An open pilot of cognitive-behavioral therapy for insomnia in women with postpartum depression. Behav Sleep Med 2013;11:297–307.

Sleep Disturbances and Suicide Risk

Rebecca A. Bernert, PhD[a],*, Michael R. Nadorff, PhD[b]

KEYWORDS

• Suicide • Psychiatric illness • Nightmares • Sleep disorders • Sleep interventions

KEY POINTS

- Suicide is a preventable public health problem that occurs in the context of psychiatric illness.
- Accounting for the presence and severity of psychopathology as a confounding variable is essential to clarifying whether disturbed sleep presents independent risk for suicidal behaviors.
- Preliminary research suggests that subjective sleep disturbances may serve as a stand-alone risk factor for suicidal ideation, attempts, and death by suicide.
- Sleep interventions appear to predict improvements in depression, and possibly suicidal ideation specifically.
- Additional research is needed to delineate poor sleep as a suicide risk factor and intervention tool for suicidal behaviors.

Suicide constitutes a global disease burden, accounting for over 1 million deaths annually. In the United States, suicide is responsible for over 30,000 fatalities every year, with an estimated 25 attempts occurring for every death by suicide.[1,2] Suicide is a complex, but preventable public health problem, with far-reaching personal and social consequences. Improvements in the identification of risk factors for suicide ultimately enhance the ability to intervene and prevent death by suicide.

Past research has identified biological, psychological, and social factors that confer elevated risk for suicide. Evidence suggests that disturbances in sleep are one such risk factor, predicting increased risk for suicidal behaviors. Both sleep disorders and general sleep complaints are linked to greater levels of suicidal ideation and depression, as well as both attempted and completed suicide.[3–6] Sleep problems are listed among the top 10 warning signs of suicide from the Substance Abuse and Mental Health Services Administration,[7] and preliminary evidence suggests that improvements in sleep may therapeutically impact depression and suicide risk.[8,9]

A REVIEW OF THE LITERATURE: IMPORTANT METHODOLOGICAL CONSIDERATIONS

Numerous investigations have evaluated sleep disturbances, such as insomnia symptoms, poor sleep quality, and nightmares, in relation to suicidal behaviors. Two methodological issues should be considered in reviewing this literature. The first issue involves the quality of methods, instruments, and measures used to assess sleep disturbance and suicidal symptoms. Early studies in this area often evaluated the relationship using only a single item to assess both sleep disturbance and suicidal symptoms, in many cases, drawn retrospectively from a brief depression inventory; yet rigorous, state-of-the-art assessment techniques exist for sleep difficulties (ie, objective sleep measures and validated symptom inventories) and suicide risk (ie, empirically based clinician-administered

[a] Department of Psychiatry and Behavioral Sciences, Stanford University School of Medicine, 401 Quarry Road, Stanford, CA 94304-5797, USA; [b] Department of Psychology, Mississippi State University, PO Box 6161, Mississippi State, MS 39762, USA
* Corresponding author.
E-mail address: rbernert@stanford.edu

Sleep Med Clin 10 (2015) 35–39
http://dx.doi.org/10.1016/j.jsmc.2014.11.004
1556-407X/15/$ – see front matter © 2015 Elsevier Inc. All rights reserved.

scales and multidimensional symptom severity instruments). The second issue involves the tendency not to adjust for the presence of psychopathology. The presence and severity of psychopathology are important potential confounders in this relationship. Suicide occurs in the presence of psychiatric illness, and over 90% of suicide decedents will have a mental disorder at the time of death.[10] In addition, both sleep disturbances and suicidal symptoms are diagnostic features of major depression.[11] Prospective investigations that utilize validated symptom measures and adjust for existing psychopathology best clarify whether poor sleep is an independent risk factor for suicide outcomes, or a mere correlate of greater psychopathology. In this article, articles have been selected and reviewed with these criteria in mind. It is organized by reports examining subjectively measured versus objectively measured sleep disturbance, and reviewed according to the type of suicidal risk evaluated (suicide ideation, suicide attempts, and suicide death).

INSOMNIA SYMPTOMS, NIGHTMARES, AND SLEEP BREATHING DISTURBANCES
Risk for Suicidal Ideation

Several investigations have examined the relationship between sleep disturbances and risk for suicidal ideation. Cukrowicz and colleagues[12] examined nightmare symptoms and suicidal ideation among a nonclinical sample of 220 undergraduate students. Insomnia and nightmare symptoms were associated with suicidal ideation, but after controlling for depression severity, only nightmares were independently associated with elevated suicidal ideation. Bernert and colleagues[13] examined self-reported sleep complaints and suicidality in a cross-sectional study of 176 psychiatric outpatients. After controlling for the influence of depression severity and other demographic factors, the association between nightmares and suicidal ideation remained significant, whereas the link between other sleep complaints (ie, insomnia and sleep-disordered breathing symptoms) and suicidality did not. Nadorff and colleagues[14] built upon this finding by evaluating insomnia and nightmares using the same self-reported symptom inventories among a nonclinical sample of 583 undergraduate students. Results again revealed that only nightmares were associated with suicidal ideation independent of symptoms of depression, anxiety, and post-traumatic stress disorder (PTSD). These findings converge somewhat with adolescent investigations. A study by Roberts and colleagues showed that, unlike the previously mentioned reports, insomnia was a significant predictor of elevated suicidal ideation with depression as a covariate.[15] A large (N = 1362) school-based survey study in China revealed that only nightmares were significantly associated with suicidal ideation after controlling for depressive symptoms.[16] Taken together, these data suggest convergence with regard to nightmares as a unique predictor of suicidal ideation. The link between insomnia and suicidal ideation remains inconsistent.

Only 1 investigation has evaluated potential sleep breathing disorders in this relationship. Krakow and colleagues[3] examined subjective sleep disturbances in 153 female sexual assault survivors with PTSD. Each woman completed various questionnaires of sleep breathing disturbances, depressive symptoms, and suicidal ideation. Participants were originally recruited for a nightmare treatment program, which may have inflated the prevalence of other co-occurring sleep complaints. Nonetheless, results indicated that women who experienced a potential sleep breathing disorder also suffered significantly greater levels of depression and suicidal ideation. Unfortunately, this study did not control for the severity of depression in this relationship to evaluate independent effects of such sleep breathing disturbances on suicide risk.

Risk for Suicide Attempts

Insomnia and nightmare symptoms also appear to serve as risk factors for overt suicidal behavior. Hall, Platt, and Hall[17] retrospectively examined the sleep of 100 consecutive patients who made suicide attempts, finding that 64% self-reported sleep onset, sleep maintenance, and terminal insomnia, and 92% reported having at least one of the three. These rates of insomnia appear disproportionately high compared with those in the general population, suggesting that complaints of insomnia may be more prevalent in those who attempt suicide than in the general public. This study did not, however, adjust for covariates to determine whether greater insomnia symptoms were explained by higher depression severity among those with a suicide attempt history.

Using a similar study design, Sjostrom and colleagues[18] retrospectively evaluated nightmares among those with a past history of suicide attempts. Results revealed that participants with nightmares had significantly higher scores on a measure of suicide risk than those without nightmares. In a subsequent study conducted by the same group, this sample was followed prospectively for 2 years.[19] Results revealed that the presence of persistent nightmares significantly predicted risk for future suicide attempts across the 2-year timeline. Even after accounting for effects of Diagnostic and Statistical

Manual of Mental Disorders axis 1 disorders including depression, anxiety, PTSD, and substance abuse, risk for a suicide attempt was approximately 4 times higher among those with persistent nightmares compared with those without.

Risk for Death by Suicide

Insomnia symptoms have also been associated with death by suicide. Fawcett and colleagues conducted one of the first studies to prospectively examine sleep, depression, and suicide.[4] In a group of depressed patients, symptoms of global insomnia were more severe among those who died by suicide within a 13-month period, suggesting insomnia symptoms may be considered a clinical indicator of acute suicidal risk. Similar findings were demonstrated in a population-based study conducted in Japan. Fujino and colleagues[5] showed that, among 13,259 middle-aged adults, only sleep maintenance insomnia at baseline, compared with other sleep disturbances (eg, difficulty initiating sleep, nonrestorative sleep), significantly predicted death by suicide 14 years later. Nevertheless, only 2 known studies have adjusted for psychopathology in assessing insomnia disturbance as a risk factor for death by suicide. First, a recent follow-up of the Nord-Trondelag Health Survey (HUNT) I study[20] found that those who endorsed insomnia disturbance nearly every night increased risk of suicide two-fold after controlling for effects of depression, anxiety, and substance abuse. Next, a psychological autopsy study of 140 adolescent suicide victims showed that, compared with 131 matched community controls, adolescent suicide decedents were 7 times more likely to exhibit insomnia symptoms (10 times for any sleep disturbance) in the week prior to death.[21] In this study, overall sleep disturbances remained a significant risk factor for death by suicide, controlling for the differential rate of affective disorder between decedents and controls, and after accounting for depression severity.

Nightmares have also been linked to death by suicide. In a prospective, population-based study conducted in Finland, Tanskanen and colleagues[6] revealed an association between nightmare frequency at baseline and completed suicides at follow-up 14 years later. Compared with subjects reporting no nightmares, those reporting occasional nightmares were 57% more likely to die by suicide, and those with frequent nightmares were 105% more likely to die by suicide. Although these findings converge with those reported for insomnia, neither study assessed for the presence of psychiatric disorders or symptoms as covariates.

Summary

In summary, multiple studies indicate that self-reported insomnia symptoms may confer independent risk for suicidal ideation, suicide attempts, and death by suicide[15,19–21]; whereas several other reports do not.[12–14] Both cross-sectional and prospective investigations suggest that nightmare symptoms are an independent risk for suicidal ideation and suicide attempts, whereas no study has evaluated the unique association between nightmares and risk for suicide death.

ELECTROENCEPHALOGRAM SLEEP STUDIES
Risk for Suicidal Ideation

Few investigations have evaluated suicide risk in association with an objective measurement of sleep. Agargun and Cartwright[22] investigated the relationship between rapid eye movement (REM) sleep, dream variables, and suicidality in depression. Compared with nonsuicidal participants, suicidal patients averaged a shorter REM sleep latency, a higher REM percentage, and a more negative dream-like quality of REM. This study did not control for depression severity, and used a single item to assess suicidal ideation. Nevertheless, abnormalities in REM would appear consistent with literature showing associations between suicidal ideation and self-reported nightmares.[13,14,16]

Risk for Suicide Attempts

Regarding risk for suicide attempts, Sabo and colleagues[23] compared depressed patients with and without a history of suicide attempts in a retrospective analysis of sleep architecture. Electroencephalographic sleep studies revealed that depressed participants with a prior suicide attempt had lower sleep efficiency, longer sleep latency, and fewer late-night delta counts. Only 1 study in this area has assessed the connection between suicidal ideation and sleep complaints beyond that explained by depression. Keshavan and colleagues[24] examined REM sleep in psychotic patients with and without a history of suicide attempts or ideation. Patients with a history of suicidal behavior showed more REM activity, and REM sleep parameters were not correlated with depression scores. Also, when depression ratings were covaried out, these differences in sleep remained.

Risk for Death by Suicide

To the authors' knowledge, no study to date has evaluated an objective assessment of disturbed sleep and risk for death by suicide.

Summary

In summary, although the previously described findings appear to converge with those for subjective sleep disturbances, results are nonetheless limited by distinct population differences (eg, psychotic vs nonpsychotic depression), study designs (retrospective or cross-sectional), and inadequate measurement techniques (single-item assessment of suicidal ideation or sleep). Although a relationship is suggested between sleep architecture abnormalities and suicide risk, additional research addressing these methodological gaps and replicating past findings is needed.

TREATMENT IMPLICATIONS AND FUTURE DIRECTIONS

Based on the previously described findings, treatment of sleep disorders to reduce risk for depression and suicide may be a fruitful area of future research. Various reports show that sleep-focused treatments predict meaningful improvements in nonsleep outcomes, including health-related quality of life, depression, and PTSD symptoms.[24–26] For the treatment of nightmares, both controlled and uncontrolled trials support the efficacy of a behavioral nightmare therapy, Imagery Rehearsal Treatment, to reduce nightmare frequency and severity.[26–29] For the treatment of insomnia, cognitive behavioral therapy for insomnia (CBTI) is considered a first-line treatment for chronic insomnia by National Institutes of Health consensus; it appears more durable than traditional hypnotics,[30] and is associated with significant improvements in depression according to randomized trials.[8,31,32] Moreover, preliminary research from the authors' group, based on a large uncontrolled trial (N = 303 community outpatients), indicates that CBTI may result in symptom reductions in suicidal ideation.[9]

In conclusion, research provides promising evidence that sleep disturbances may confer independent risk for suicidal behaviors, and 1 preliminary finding suggests that treatment of sleep problems may decrease risk for suicide ideation. Future studies are needed, rigorous in design and methodology, to further delineate poor sleep as an independent suicide risk factor and intervention tool. Both in research and in clinical practice, the authors recommend standard use of empirically supported suicide risk assessment frameworks[33] to routine clinical decision-making and emergency referral procedures in the treatment and management of suicidal behaviors.

REFERENCES

1. Krug EG, Dahlberg L, Mercy J, et al. World report on violence health. Geneva (Switzerland): World Health Organization; 2002.
2. Centers for Disease Control and Prevention. Web-based injury statistics query and reporting system. 2011. Available at: http://www.cdc.gov/injury/wisqars/index.html. Accessed October 15, 2011.
3. Krakow B, Artar A, Warner TD, et al. Sleep disorder, depression and suicidality in female sexual assault survivors. Crisis 2000;21(4):163–70.
4. Fawcett J, Scheftner WA, Fogg L, et al. Time-related predictors of suicide in major affective disorder. Am J Psychiatry 1990;147(9):1189–94.
5. Fujino Y, Mizoue T, Tokui N, et al. Prospective cohort study of stress, life satisfaction, self-rated health, insomnia, and suicide death in Japan. Suicide Life Threat Behav 2005;35(2):227–37.
6. Tanskanen A, Tuomilehto J, Viinamäki H, et al. Nightmares as predictors of suicide. Sleep 2001;24(7):844–7.
7. National Mental Health Information Center. Suicide warning signs [Internet]. Substance Abuse and Mental Health Services Administration (SAMHSA). 2005. Available at: http://www.mentalhealth.samhsa.gov/publications/allpubs/walletcard/engwalletcard.asp. Accessed November 5, 2006.
8. Buysse DJ, Germain A, Moul DE, et al. Efficacy of a brief behavioral treatment for chronic insomnia in older adults. Arch Intern Med 2011;171(10):887–95.
9. Manber R, Bernert RA, Suh S, et al. CBT for insomnia in patients with high and low depressive symptom severity: adherence and clinical outcomes. J Clin Sleep Med 2012;7(6):645–52.
10. Bertolote JM, Fleischmann A, De Leo D, et al. Psychiatric diagnoses and suicide: revisiting the evidence. Crisis 2004;25(4):147–55.
11. The Diagnostic and Statistical Manual of Mental Disorders. 4th edition. Text revision. Washington, DC: American Psychiatric Association; 2000.
12. Cukrowicz KC, Otamendi A, Pinto JV, et al. The impact of insomnia and sleep disturbances on depression and suicidality. Dreaming 2006;16(1):1–10.
13. Bernert RA, Joiner TE, Cukrowicz KC, et al. Suicidality and sleep disturbances. Sleep 2005;28(9):1135–41.
14. Nadorff MR, Nazem S, Fiske A. Insomnia symptoms, nightmares, and suicidal ideation in a college student sample. Sleep 2011;34(1):93–8.
15. Roberts RE, Roberts CR, Chen IG. Functioning of adolescents with symptoms of disturbed sleep. J Youth Adolesc 2001;30(1):1–18.
16. Liu X. Sleep and adolescent suicidal behavior. Sleep 2004;27:1351–8.

17. Hall RC, Platt DC, Hall RC. Suicide risk assessment: a review of risk factors for suicide in 100 patients who made severe suicide attempts. Evaluation of suicide risk in a time of managed care. Psychosomatics 1999;40(1):18–27.

18. Sjostrom NM, Waern M, Hetta J. Nightmares and sleep disturbances in relation to suicidality in suicide attempters. Sleep 2007;30(1):91–5.

19. Sjostrom NJ, Hetta J, Waern M. Persistent nightmares are associated with repeat suicide attempt: a prospective study. Psychiatry Res 2009;170(2–3):208–11.

20. Bjørngaard JH, Bjerkeset O, Romundstad P, et al. Sleeping problems and suicide in 75,000 Norwegian adults: a 20 year follow-up of the HUNT I study. Sleep 2011;34(9):1155–9.

21. Goldstein TR, Brent DA, Bridge JA. Sleep disturbance preceding completed suicide in adolescents. J Consult Clin Psychol 2008;76(1):84–91.

22. Agargun MY, Cartwright R. REM sleep, dream variables and suicidality in depressed patients. Psychiatry Res 2003;119(1–2):33–9.

23. Sabo E, Reynolds CF 3rd, Kupfer DJ, et al. Sleep, depression, and suicide. Psychiatry Res 1991; 36(3):265–77.

24. McCall WV, Blocker JN, D'Agostino R Jr, et al. Treatment of insomnia in depressed insomniacs: effects on health-related quality of life, objective and self-reported sleep, and depression. J Clin Sleep Med 2010;6(4):322–9.

25. Snedecor SJ, Botteman MF, Schaefer K, et al. Economic outcomes of eszopiclone treatment in insomnia and comorbid major depressive disorder. J Ment Health Policy Econ 2010;13(1):27–35.

26. Krakow B, Hollifeld M, Johnston L, et al. Imagery rehearsal therapy for chronic nightmares in sexual assault survivors with PTSD: a randomized controlled trial. JAMA 2001;286(5):537–45.

27. Ulmer CS, Edinger JD, Calhoun PS. A multi-component cognitive–behavioral invervention for sleep disturbance in veterans with PTSD: a pilot study. J Clin Sleep Med 2011;7(1):57–68.

28. Germain A, Nielsen TA. Impact of imagery rehearsal treatment on distressing dreams, psychological distress, and sleep parameters in nightmare patients. Behav Sleep Med 2003;1:140–54.

29. Germain A, Shear MK, Hall M, et al. Effects of a brief behavioral treatment for PTSD related sleep disturbances: a pilot study. Behav Res Ther 2007;45(3): 627–32.

30. NIH state-of-the-science conference statement on manifestations and management of chronic insomnia in adults. NIH Consens State Sci Statements 2005; 22(2):1–30.

31. Morin CM, Vallières A, Guay B, et al. Cognitive behavioral therapy, singly and combined with medication, for persistent insomnia: a randomized controlled trial. JAMA 2009;301(19):2005–15.

32. Manber R, Edinger JD, Gress JL, et al. Cognitive behavioral therapy for insomnia enhances depression outcome in patients with comorbid major depressive disorder and insomnia. Sleep 2008; 31(4):489–95.

33. Joiner TE, Walker RL, Rudd MD, et al. Scientizing and routinizing the assessment of suicidality in outpatient practice. Prof Psychol Res Pract 1990; 30(5):447–53.

Posttraumatic Stress Disorder and Sleep

Wilfred R. Pigeon, PhD, CBSM[a,b,c],*, Autumn M. Gallegos, PhD[a,b]

KEYWORDS

- Posttraumatic stress disorder • Insomnia • Cognitive-behavioral therapy for insomnia

KEY POINTS

- Sleep disturbance in general as well as several specific sleep disorders are observed at high rates among patients with posttraumatic stress disorder (PTSD).
- Nightmares are quite specific to PTSD and tend to ameliorate following standard treatments for PTSD; insomnia is more prevalent and tends to persist absent direct intervention.
- Prazosin and imagery rehearsal therapy have demonstrated efficacy for nightmares; benzodiazepine receptor agonists and cognitive-behavioral therapy for insomnia (CBT-I) have demonstrated efficacy and effectiveness for general insomnia.
- PTSD-related insomnia presents with unique features that require assessment and targeting.
- Standard CBT-I can be easily adapted to address the unique presentations of patients with PTSD and insomnia.
- Combining CBT-I with imagery rehearsal therapy is a promising approach to the nonpharmacologic management of co-occurring insomnia and nightmares in patients with PTSD.

INTRODUCTION

Sleep disturbances are a common feature of posttraumatic stress disorder (PTSD)[1] and have historically been considered the hallmark of PTSD.[2] They have been found to occur in 70% of participants meeting the diagnostic criteria for PTSD in a large-scale community survey.[1] Ample data suggest a strong association between trauma exposure and nightmares as well as between PTSD and nightmares.[3] Insomnia (difficulty initiating or maintaining sleep) is actually more prevalent than nightmares among people with PTSD and is the most commonly endorsed PTSD symptom.[4] This point underscores the specificity of nightmares for PTSD as well as the high prevalence of insomnia in trauma-exposed populations of 60% to 90% in contrast to the 6% to 20% prevalence rate in the general population.[5] Nightmares and insomnia are each independently associated with PTSD[6] and have also been found to be risk factors for developing PTSD in a handful of studies.[7–9] Finally, and quite importantly, the additional burden of insomnia and/or nightmares may directly exacerbate other PTSD symptoms and diminish patients' capacity to manage their PTSD symptoms.

Funding sources: This material is, in part, the result of work supported with resources and the use of facilities at the Center of Excellence for Suicide Prevention, VA Medical Center, Canandaigua, NY. The contents do not represent the views of the Department of Veterans Affairs or the United States Government.
Conflict of interest: nil.
a Department of Veterans Affairs VISN 2 Center of Excellence for Suicide Prevention, Canandaigua VA Medical Center, 400 Fort Hill Road, Canandaigua, NY 14424, USA; b Sleep and Neurophysiology Research Laboratory, Department of Psychiatry, University of Rochester Medical Center, 300 Crittenden Boulevard, Rochester, NY 14642, USA; c Department of Veterans Affairs Center for Integrated Healthcare, Syracuse VA Medical Center, 800 Irving Avenue, Syracuse, NY 13210, USA
* Corresponding author. Sleep and Neurophysiology Research Laboratory, Department of Psychiatry, University of Rochester Medical Center, 300 Crittenden Boulevard, Rochester, NY 14642.
E-mail address: Wilfred_Pigeon@urmc.rochester.edu

THE OBJECTIVE SLEEP OF PATIENTS WITH POSTTRAUMATIC STRESS DISORDER

Recent reviews of PTSD and sleep have concluded that the available literature is somewhat mixed with respect to polysomnography (PSG) findings in PTSD populations.[10,11] There have nonetheless been some consistent findings of note. Although evaluated in a smaller number of PSG studies, abnormalities of rapid-eye-movement (REM) sleep do seem to occur in patients with or developing PTSD. These abnormalities include increased levels of awakenings from REM and brief arousals during REM, more and shorter duration REM periods, and elevated REM density. These data suggest that beyond insomnia, the main PSG-determined characteristics of sleep in patients with PTSD are disturbances of REM sleep. Sleep disturbances, such as sleep-disordered breathing (eg, sleep apnea), parasomnias, and excessive nocturnal motor activity (eg, periodic limb movements), have been reported in PTSD populations[10,12,13]; but the primary focus of this article is on nightmares and insomnia and on nonpharmacologic interventions for these sleep disorders.

THE NATURE OF INSOMNIA AND NIGHTMARES IN POSTTRAUMATIC STRESS DISORDER

PTSD-related insomnia is similar to primary insomnia along several dimensions, including the subjective severity of insomnia and the association with a higher risk for other complications.[6,14-18] It is important to note that these findings come from a relatively small number of studies with small to modest sample sizes across a variety of civilian and combat-related PTSD populations. Nonetheless, the implications are that PTSD-related insomnia is similar to primary insomnia in many regards with the possibility that any increased severity is caused by additional disturbances that occur during sleep and/or are unique to patients with PTSD.

There is strong evidence that patients with insomnia exhibit hyperarousal across several dimensions, including physiologic and cognitive indices of arousal that interfere with sleep and thought to be a precipitant of insomnia.[19] Most theoretic models of chronic insomnia include the notion that, once acute insomnia has been precipitated, many of the same factors continue to maintain or perpetuate insomnia and that these are further exacerbated by behavioral factors commonly observed in insomnia. It is possible, and indeed likely, that some of these factors may

be exacerbated in PTSD-related insomnia and that additional factors may further distinguish patients with PTSD.

In PTSD-related insomnia, the traumatic event serves to create a state level of arousal (cognitive and/or physiologic), which can then precipitate insomnia (or worsen/maintain preexisting insomnia). Morin and Espie[20] proposed that reactive anxiety (a central element of PTSD) is the main contributing factor in the acute phase of insomnia. Thus, the traumatic events and ongoing stressor of having PTSD are themselves unique features of PTSD-related insomnia. Patients with insomnia with PTSD (as opposed to those without PTSD) have significantly more fear of sleep, fear of the dark, disturbing thoughts in bed, daytime fatigue, and anxiety.

Perceived loss of control, which is thought to contribute to the maintenance of PTSD,[21] may also be exacerbated in the acute period following a traumatic event as sleep becomes disrupted and individuals attempt typically counterproductive strategies to control sleep. Because sleep itself involves a loss of vigilance and the restricted ability to monitor one's environment, sleep may be further perceived as a loss of control and/or something to fear.[22] For individuals with PTSD, fear and vigilance may lead to particular sleep behaviors and cognitions, such as the use of heavy blankets to feel safe (which may elevate body temperature and disrupt sleep), and exaggerated safety behaviors, such as securing and checking the sleep environment (which is also counterproductive to sleep). Finally, sleep itself can be directly related to fear experienced during a trauma. Patients with a history of being traumatized in bed, the bedroom, or darkness are more likely to report insomnia after successfully completing cognitive-behavioral therapy (CBT) for PTSD.[23] In sum, these represent distinct features of insomnia not typically observed in patients without PTSD.

Nightmares also represent a unique feature of PTSD-related insomnia. Although insomnia is more prevalent than nightmares in PTSD, nightmares seldom occur in the absence of insomnia and may contribute to the development or maintenance of insomnia in PTSD.[24] Nightmare sufferers, in general, delay going to bed or returning to bed following nightmares. To the extent that presleep anxiety develops because of nightmares, this serves to reduce the likelihood of initiating sleep. Nightmares are arousing and make returning to sleep difficult; as replays of traumatic experiences, nightmares can elicit and reinforce the same fear and avoidance responses as the original trauma, providing an avenue to associate sleep with the anxiety and fear experienced during nightmares.[25]

Moreover, nightmares may have a negative impact on the ability to process emotional information by disrupting sleep in general and REM sleep specifically.[26] Taken together, the sleep disturbance inherent in nightmares and insomnia can promote or exacerbate negative emotions for patients with PTSD, including irritability, anxiety, and depression, while diminishing the capacity to process or cope with such emotions.

STANDARD TREATMENTS OF POSTTRAUMATIC STRESS DISORDER AND THEIR EFFECT ON SLEEP

Although effective pharmacologic and psychotherapeutic interventions for PTSD exist, they devote little focused attention to directly improving sleep. Indeed, available data suggest limited efficacy of standard psychological and pharmacologic.[23,27–31] PTSD treatments on insomnia, making sleep disturbance one of the most common residual symptoms of remitted PTSD. In general, insomnia persists robustly without direct intervention[32] and, importantly, in the presence of insomnia, PTSD is less likely to remit than in the absence of sleep problems.[33] In the context of PTSD, the need for direct sleep interventions is well founded.

STANDARD TREATMENTS FOR INSOMNIA AND NIGHTMARES

Based on several meta-analyses and the extant literature for benzodiazepines, benzodiazepine receptor agonists (BZRAs), and CBT for insomnia (CBT-I), a 2005 National Institutes of Health State of the Science Conference[34] concluded that BZRAs and CBT-I are effective to treat insomnia in the short-term with relatively benign side-effect profiles and that CBT-I has more durable effects when active treatment is discontinued. Both modes of treatment have demonstrated consistently large effect sizes, although CBT-I is indicated for chronic insomnia and in acute insomnia in individuals for whom pharmacotherapy is contraindicated.

Two approaches to treat nightmares are supported by a growing evidence base. Prazosin, which was originally introduced to treat hypertension, is a short-acting nonsedating generic alpha-1 adrenoreceptor antagonist that easily crosses the blood-brain barrier. In addition to positive findings in case series, retrospective chart reviews, and some small open label trials, prazosin has been found to markedly reduce nightmares and sleep disturbance in 3 placebo-controlled trials: 2 in Vietnam veterans and one in a civilian PTSD cohort.[35–37]

Imagery rehearsal therapy (IRT), a term the authors use here to refer to cognitive and/or behavioral techniques focusing on altering dream content, has also been used to successfully treat nightmares in more than a dozen investigations with large to very large effect sizes for nightmare frequency and intensity and gains maintained for up to 6 months.[38] Like prazosin, the improvements in nightmares have also been found to generalize to overall sleep quality,[38] although no effect of IRT on nightmares, compared with an active control condition, was observed in a randomized trial in Vietnam veterans.[39] Unlike with the use of prazosin for nightmares, there is no return of nightmares following discontinuation of IRT in the short-term. Both IRT and prazosin seem effective for nightmares with some associated improvements for insomnia and for PTSD. Thus, effective interventions do exist for the two most common forms of sleep disturbance in PTSD, insomnia and nightmares. Again, this article focuses on the nonpharmacologic interventions in more detail.

COGNITIVE-BEHAVIORAL THERAPY FOR INSOMNIA

Standard CBT-I is composed of several specific psychotherapeutic interventions that draw on cognitive therapy and behavioral therapy as they are applied to insomnia. The individual components may be delivered as monotherapies, although it is widely accepted that multicomponent CBT-I is the best approach to treatment, addressing the multiple putative causes and perpetuators of insomnia. The components of therapy include sleep education, stimulus control, sleep restriction (**Box 1**), sleep hygiene, cognitive therapy, and relaxation therapy. CBT-I is typically structured to allow for weekly sessions over 6 to 8 weeks in group or individual therapy, although CBT-I delivered in 2 to 4 sessions has demonstrated good efficacy. In the clinical setting, the number of sessions can be altered based on treatment progress and the patients' ability to self-administer (and monitor) the interventions.

Cognitive-Behavioral Therapy for Insomnia Overview

Sleep education
Sleep education consists of providing patients with a basic knowledge about sleep processes and functions, sleep architecture, developmental changes in sleep, circadian rhythms, individual sleep needs, and sleep deprivation. Sleep education also often comprises providing a treatment rationale, setting treatment expectations, and establishing motivation for treatment.

Box 1
Behavioral components of CBT-I

Stimulus Control

1. Limit the amount of time spent awake in bed or the bedroom
2. Keep fixed wake time 7 days per week
3. Avoid behavior in the bed or bedroom other than sleep or sexual activity
4. Sleep only in the bedroom
5. Leave the bedroom when awake for approximately 15 to 20 minutes
6. Return to the bed only when sleepy

Sleep Restriction

1. Limit the amount of time spent in bed to an amount equal to their average total sleep time
2. Establish an average total sleep time (TST) from 1 to 2 weeks of daily sleep diaries
3. Establish a fixed wake time
4. Establish a sleep window by setting bedtime to allow for total sleep opportunity equal to TST from prior diaries (do not set sleep window less than 5 hours even if TST is shorter than this amount)
5. Continue to keep weekly sleep diaries
6. Adjust the sleep window based on weekly sleep efficiency derived from the prior weeks' sleep diaries (eg, if sleep efficiency (TST/sleep window) is greater than or equal to 90% (some use 85% as the benchmark), increase sleep window by 15 minutes
7. Continue daily sleep diaries and adjustments on a weekly basis until treatment completion

The two main behavioral components of CBT-I (and perhaps the most active components of the intervention) are stimulus control and sleep restriction therapy (see **Box 1**).

Sleep hygiene

Sleep hygiene requires that the clinician and patients review a set of instructions that are geared toward helping patients maintain good sleep habits, such as keeping an environment and routine conducive to sleep, maintaining a regular bed and wake time, and avoiding tobacco, alcohol, large meals, and vigorous exercise for several hours before bed.

Cognitive therapy

Cognitive therapy for insomnia has been developed in a few forms that often overlap. Some have a more didactic focus, whereas others use paradoxic intention, cognitive restructuring, modification of safety behaviors, and/or attentional biases. Although the approaches differ in procedure, all are based on the observation that patients with insomnia have negative thoughts and beliefs about their condition and its consequences. Helping patients to challenge the veracity and usefulness of these beliefs is the basis of cognitive therapy and is thought to decrease the anxiety and arousal associated with insomnia.

Relaxation training

Relaxation training may also proceed with one or more relaxation techniques, including progressive muscle relaxation, diaphragmatic breathing, biofeedback, and more formal meditative techniques to decrease overall hyperarousal. The optimal relaxation method for insomnia is the technique that is most acceptable to and/or easiest to learn for patients. Some techniques may be contraindicated by medical conditions (eg, progressive muscle relaxation might not be ideal for patients with chronic pain conditions, which can be quite prevalent in the veteran population) or psychiatric disorders (eg, some techniques are difficult for patients with untreated PTSD to tolerate as they can precipitate re-experiencing symptoms).

IMAGERY REHEARSAL THERAPY

IRT refers to treatments that use cognitive and/or behavioral techniques to treat nightmares. The first technique is based on exposure therapy in which patients are asked to describe a distressing dream and to rehearse it. (In some versions of this approach, the dream is written down and rehearsed.) The second technique is based loosely on cognitive restructuring in which patients are asked to change something about the dream content and to rehearse this changed dream. An expanded variant of IRT, called *exposure, relaxation, and rescripting therapy*, consists of the combination of education about trauma, PTSD, and sleep; exposure to the nightmare content and distressing themes during the session; diaphragmatic breathing; daily progressive muscle relaxation; promotion of healthy sleep practices; and rescripting of the nightmare scenario guided by therapists and group members.

Although nightmare exposure alone can be effective, most versions of IRT direct patients to change part of their nightmare narrative and to mentally rehearse the new dream while making it as vivid as possible. Practitioners of IRT vary on what they tell their patients to change (ie, the dream ending, the most disturbing feature of the dream, or anything in the dream). Thus, applications of IRT also vary in the extent to which the treatment involves exposure to traumatic images/memories. Other features can also vary, including the length of treatment (although typically it ranges from 1–6 face-to-face sessions), whether delivered individually or in groups, the extent of between-session practice, and the dream that is the focus of treatment (eg, a nightmare that reflects the actual traumatic event, the worst nightmare, a nightmare that is less threatening, and so forth). Clinical experience to date suggests that changing anything in the dream is as effective as any other approach, that avoiding focusing on a nightmare that is exactly trauma replicating is preferred, and that the dream need not be at all related to the actual trauma. In general, the available literature suggests that IRT and its variants may be associated with clinically meaningful improvements in nightmares and that it has high tolerability and safety.

TAILORING COGNITIVE-BEHAVIORAL THERAPY FOR INSOMNIA FOR PATIENTS WITH POSTTRAUMATIC STRESS DISORDER

PTSD-related insomnia, which may follow a similar course as other comorbid insomnias, is nonetheless maintained by features that are unique to or accentuated in trauma populations. These features, in turn, provide clinically relevant targets for intervention that may also be unique to insomnia in patients with PTSD. Tailoring CBT-I for patients with PTSD begins by enhancing the assessment of unique thoughts and behaviors that may be present in this population. Specifically, assessment should include questions pertaining to sleep avoidance, fear of sleep, and nocturnal vigilance; asking whether traumatic events occurred during sleep or in a sleep environment; and determining to what extent nightmares are occurring and disrupting sleep. This assessment entails identifying behaviors that may interfere with sleep initiation (eg, excessive safety checking or using alcohol to fall asleep) and cognitions that are maladaptive and/or increase cognitive arousal (eg, sleeping is not safe).

Based on what is learned during assessment, both cognitions and behaviors can be addressed in the course of standard CBT-I. For instance, behaviors that interfere with sleep can be targeted for modification as part of stimulus control or sleep hygiene. Maladaptive cognition, in turn, can be addressed during cognitive therapy modules. Sleep education may also be enhanced to include information about the interaction of PTSD and

sleep problems and the futility of avoiding sleep to avoid nightmares given that sleep deprivation leads to REM rebound and more intense dreaming. As noted, if relaxation training is to be used, it may be useful to avoid relaxation strategies that may lead to re-experiencing symptoms. To the extent that nightmares are present and problematic, they most likely need to be addressed in more depth.

COMBINING COGNITIVE-BEHAVIORAL THERAPY FOR INSOMNIA AND IMAGERY REHEARSAL THERAPY

When PTSD-related insomnia coexists with nightmares that are contributing to sleep disturbance, CBT-I may be combined with IRT (Fig. 1). The two approaches have been combined with promising results in veterans with PTSD. Ulmer and colleagues[40] compared such a combined treatment approach (n = 8) to treatment as usual (n = 9). Treatment was delivered in 6 individual biweekly sessions. Statistically significant and large effects for the combined intervention were observed on sleep outcomes in addition to an approximately 30% decrease in PTSD severity but without an observed effect on depression. Another clinical trial randomized veterans with chronic sleep disturbance to receive a behavioral sleep intervention that combined IRT with stimulus control and sleep restriction (n = 17; see Box 1), prazosin (n = 18), or a placebo (n = 15). Both active treatments significantly reduced insomnia severity and PTSD symptoms after 8 weeks of intervention.[41] A combined version of IRT and CBT for insomnia was also delivered in an uncontrolled 10-session group therapy intervention (n = 10) with moderate to large effect sizes for nightmares and insomnia[42] and in a separate uncontrolled trial[43] to combat veterans (n = 15) over 8 individual sessions with large to very large effects on insomnia and nightmares along with a moderate to large effect for PTSD and depression severity.

Although limited to 3 small randomized trials and 2 uncontrolled pilot studies, these data suggest that combining cognitive-behavioral treatment of insomnia and nightmares in populations exposed to trauma is feasible, efficacious, and warrants replication. Whether gains in sleep improvements generalize to clinically meaningful attenuation of mental health symptoms is an ongoing empirical question. However, given that there does seem to be some reduction in PTSD severity, this raises the possibility that CBT-I and/or IRT might also be combined with or sequenced with standard PTSD treatments for maximal effect.

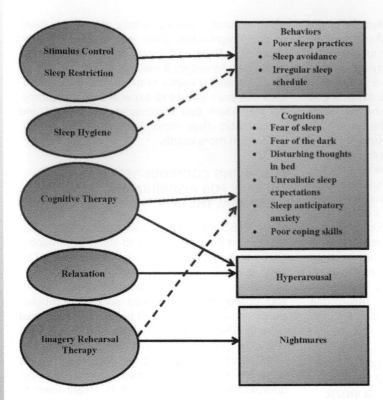

Fig. 1. A diagram of how components of combined CBT-I and IRT address typical and PTSD-related features of insomnia. The circles represent components of combined cognitive-behavioral treatments for insomnia and nightmares; the blocks represent common manifestations of PTSD-related insomnia; arrows indicate the targets of each intervention, with dotted lines indicating targets that are more speculative.

SUMMARY

Patients with PTSD have high rates of sleep disturbance in general as well as several specific sleep disorders. Nightmares are specific to PTSD and are effectively treated with prazosin and IRT, whereas BZRAs and CBT-I demonstrate efficacy and effectiveness for general insomnia. PTSD-related insomnia presents unique features that require assessment and targeting, and standard CBT-I can be adapted to address these issues. Combining CBT-I and IRT is a promising approach to nonpharmacologic management of co-occurring insomnia and nightmares in patients with PTSD.

REFERENCES

1. Ohayon MM, Shapiro CM. Sleep disturbances and psychiatric disorders associated with posttraumatic stress disorder in the general population. Compr Psychiatry 2000;41:469–78.

2. Ross RJ, Ball WA, Sullivan KA, et al. Sleep disturbances as the hallmark of posttraumatic stress disorder. Am J Psychiatry 1989;146:697–707.

3. Mellman TA, Pigeon WR. Dreams and nightmares in posttraumatic stress disorder. In: Kryger M, Roth T, Dement WC, editors. Principles and practice of sleep medicine. 4th edition. Philadelphia: Elsevier Saunders; 2005. p. 573–8.

4. Green BL. Disasters and posttraumatic stress disorder. In: Davidson JR, Foa EB, editors. Posttraumatic stress disorder: DSM-IV and beyond. Washington, DC: American Psychiatric Press; 1993. p. 75–97.

5. Ohayon MM. Epidemiology of insomnia: what we know and what we still need to learn. Sleep Med Rev 2002;6:97–111.

6. Clum GA, Nishith P, Resick PA. Trauma-related sleep disturbance and self-reported physical health symptoms in treatment-seeking female rape victims. J Nerv Ment Dis 2001;189:618–22.

7. Harvey AG, Bryant RA. The relationship between acute stress disorder and posttraumatic stress disorder: a prospective evaluation of motor vehicle accident survivors. J Consult Clin Psychol 1998; 66:507–12.

8. Mellman TA, Pigeon WR, Nowell PD, et al. Relationships between REM sleep findings and PTSD symptoms during the early aftermath of trauma. J Trauma Stress 2007;20:893–901.

9. Koren D, Arnon I, Lavie P, et al. Sleep complaints as early predictors of posttraumatic stress disorder: a 1-year prospective study of injured survivors of motor vehicle accidents. Am J Psychiatry 2002;159: 855–7.

10. Spoormaker VI, Montgomery P. Disturbed sleep in post-traumatic stress disorder: secondary symptom or core feature? Sleep Med Rev 2008;12:169–84.

11. Germain A, Buysse DJ, Nofzinger E. Sleep-specific mechanisms underlying posttraumatic stress disorder: integrative review and neurobiological hypotheses. Sleep Med Rev 2008;12:185–95.

12. Krakow B, Melendrez D, Pedersen B, et al. Complex insomnia: insomnia and sleep-disordered breathing in a consecutive series of crime victims with nightmares and PTSD. Biol Psychiatry 2001;49:948–53.

13. Germain A, Nielsen TA. Sleep pathophysiology in posttraumatic stress disorder and idiopathic nightmare sufferers. Biol Psychiatry 2003;54:1092–8.

14. Woodward SH, Bliwise DL, Friedman MJ, et al. Subjective versus objective sleep in Vietnam combat veterans hospitalized for PTSD. J Trauma Stress 1996;9:137–43.

15. Mellman TA, Kulick-Bell R, Ashlock LE, et al. Sleep events among veterans with combat-related posttraumatic stress disorder. Am J Psychiatry 1995;152:110–5.

16. Nishith P, Resick PA, Mueser KT. Sleep difficulties and alcohol use motives in female rape victims with posttraumatic stress disorder. J Trauma Stress 2001;14:469–79.

17. Calhoun PS, Wiley M, Dennis MF, et al. Objective evidence of sleep disturbance in women with posttraumatic stress disorder. J Trauma Stress 2007;20:1009–18.

18. Inman DJ, Silver S, Doghramji K. Sleep disturbance in post-traumatic stress disorder: a comparison with non-PTSD insomnia. J Trauma Stress 1990;3:429–37.

19. Perlis M, Smith MT, Pigeon W. The etiology and pathophysiology of primary insomnia. In: Kryger M, Roth T, Dement W, editors. Principles and practice of sleep medicine. 4th edition. Philadelphia: W.B. Saunders Company; 2005. p. 714–25.

20. Morin CM, Espie CA. Insomnia: a clinical guide to assessment and treatment. New York: Kluwer Academic/Plenum Press; 2003.

21. Ehlers A, Hackmann A, Michael T. Intrusive re-experiencing in post-traumatic stress disorder: phenomenology, theory, and therapy. Memory 2004;12:403–15.

22. Craske MG, Tsao JC. Assessment and treatment of nocturnal panic attacks. Sleep Med Rev 2005;9:173–84.

23. Zayfert C, Deviva JC. Residual insomnia following cognitive behavioral therapy for PTSD. J Trauma Stress 2004;17:69–73.

24. Kobayashi I, Sledjeski EM, Spoonster E, et al. Effects of early nightmares on the development of sleep disturbances in motor vehicle accident victims. J Trauma Stress 2008;21:548–55.

25. Mellman TA. Sleep and the pathogenesis of PTSD. International handbook of human response to trauma. New York: Plenum Press; 2000.

26. Stickgold R. Sleep-dependent memory consolidation. Nature 2005;437:1272–8.

27. Lamarche LJ, De Koninck J. Sleep disturbance in adults with posttraumatic stress disorder: a review. J Clin Psychiatry 2007;68:1257–70.

28. Lange A, Rietdijk D, Hudcovicova M, et al. Interapy: a controlled randomized trial of the standardized treatment of posttraumatic stress through the Internet. J Consult Clin Psychol 2003;71:901–9.

29. Galovski TE, Monson C, Bruce SE, et al. Does cognitive-behavioral therapy for PTSD improve perceived health and sleep impairment? J Trauma Stress 2009;22:197–204.

30. Belleville G, Guay S, Marchand A. Persistence of sleep disturbances following cognitive-behavior therapy for posttraumatic stress disorder. J Psychosom Res 2011;70:318–27.

31. Stein DJ, Davidson J, Seedat S, et al. Paroxetine in the treatment of post-traumatic stress disorder: pooled analysis of placebo-controlled studies. Expert Opin Pharmacother 2003;4:1829–38.

32. Mendelson WB. Long-term follow-up of chronic insomnia. Sleep 1995;18:698–701.

33. Marcks BA, Weisberg RB, Edelen MO, et al. The relationship between sleep disturbance and the course of anxiety disorders in primary care patients. Psychiatry Res 2010;178:487–92.

34. Leshner AI, Baghdoyan HA, Bennett SJ. National Institutes of Health State-of-the-Science Conference Statement on Manifestations and Management of Chronic Insomnia in Adults (final statement). Sleep 2005;28:1049–57.

35. Raskind MA, Peskind ER, Kanter ED, et al. Reduction of nightmares and other PTSD symptoms in combat veterans by prazosin: a placebo-controlled study. Am J Psychiatry 2003;160:371–3.

36. Raskind MA, Peskind ER, Hoff DJ, et al. A parallel group placebo controlled study of prazosin for trauma nightmares and sleep disturbance in combat veterans with post-traumatic stress disorder. Biol Psychiatry 2007;61:928–34.

37. Taylor FB, Martin P, Thompson C, et al. Prazosin effects on objective sleep measures and clinical symptoms in civilian trauma PTSD: a placebo-controlled study. Biol Psychiatry 2008;63:629–32.

38. Lancee J, Spoormaker VI, Krakow B, et al. A systematic review of cognitive-behavioral treatment for nightmares: toward a well-established treatment. J Clin Sleep Med 2008;4:475–80.

39. Cook JM, Harb GC, Gehrman PR, et al. Imagery rehearsal for posttraumatic nightmares: a randomized controlled trial. J Trauma Stress 2010;23:553–63.

40. Ulmer CS, Edinger JD, Calhoun PS. A multi-component cognitive-behavioral intervention for sleep

disturbance in veterans with PTSD: a pilot study. J Clin Sleep Med 2011;7:57–68.

41. Germain A, Richardson R, Moul DE, et al. Placebo-controlled comparison of prazosin and cognitive-behavioral treatments for sleep disturbances in US military veterans. J Psychosom Res 2012;72: 89–96.

42. Swanson LM, Favorite TK, Horin E, et al. A combined group treatment for nightmares and insomnia in combat veterans: a pilot study. J Trauma Stress 2009;22:639–42.

43. Pigeon WR, Matteson-Rusby SE, Claassen C, et al. CBT for sleep disturbances in combat veterans: preliminary findings. Sleep 2010;33S:A236.

Sleep in Schizophrenia
Pathology and Treatment

Kathleen L. Benson, PhD[a,b,]*

KEYWORDS

- Schizophrenia • Sleep • Insomnia • Polysomnography • Side effects • Sleep disorders

KEY POINTS

- Insomnia is a hallmark of schizophrenia, and a marked increase in insomnia is a prodromal sign of impending psychosis or clinical relapse.
- In general, antipsychotic agents (APs) ameliorate this insomnia.
- However, APs may also induce or exacerbate comorbid sleep disorders such as restless legs syndrome or sleep-disordered breathing.
- Sleep disorders in schizophrenia should be vigorously treated.
- A positive clinical outcome may be associated with the normalization of sleep and its restorative processes.

SCHIZOPHRENIA: A BRIEF OVERVIEW

Our understanding of schizophrenia continues to advance in a range of diverse disciplines: psychiatry, genetics, neurology, physiology, biochemistry, pharmacology, pathology, and epidemiology. Although the etiology of the disease presents an ongoing challenge, the prevailing model to emerge views schizophrenia as a neurodevelopmental disorder with a lifetime prevalence of 0.7% and a male-to-female incidence ratio of 1.4 worldwide.[1]

Despite decades of research, there is no laboratory-based diagnostic specific to schizophrenia. The diagnosis remains a clinical entity, and the American Psychiatric Association is the recognized source of the current diagnostic criteria published as the DSM-5 (*Diagnostic and Statistical Manual of Mental Disorders*, 5th edition).[2] These defining criteria of schizophrenia encompass 2 categories: positive symptoms and negative symptoms. Positive symptoms include hallucinations and delusions (a psychotic dimension) in addition to disorganized speech and catatonic behavior (a disorganized dimension). Negative symptoms include affective

flattening, avolition, and poverty of speech. Additional criteria include marked deterioration in occupational and social functioning. Furthermore, the diagnosis of schizophrenia must exclude psychotic disturbances attributable to a variety of medical, psychiatric, and substance abuse disorders. The early onset and subsequent course of illness, along with clinical outcome studies, suggest that schizophrenia is likely the most devastating of all psychiatric illnesses, which can be neither prevented nor cured. Most schizophrenics, particularly after an early onset, experience long-term mental disability, higher rates of morbidity and mortality, and social and economic marginalization.

Risk factors associated with the development of schizophrenia include both genetic and environmental factors, with genetic heritability estimated at 81%.[3] Thus, genetic makeup alone is not sufficient for the development of schizophrenia, and an array of environmental factors, both prenatal and postnatal, have been suggested as contributory factors. In part, current research focuses on the role of epigenetic mechanisms that could

Disclosure: This was not an industry-supported study. There is no financial conflict of interest.
[a] Neuroimaging Section, McLean Hospital, 115 Milk Street, Belmont, MA 02478, USA; [b] Department of Psychiatry, Harvard Medical School, 401 Park Drive, Boston, MA 02215, USA
* PO Box 335, Barnstable, MA 02630.
E-mail address: kbenson@mclean.harvard.edu

Sleep Med Clin 10 (2015) 49–55
http://dx.doi.org/10.1016/j.jsmc.2014.11.001
1556-407X/15/$ – see front matter © 2015 Elsevier Inc. All rights reserved.

mediate the interaction of environment and gene expression.[4] Multiple genetic, epigenetic, and environmental factors are consistent with the diverse range of expressed phenotypes, and are consistent with the notion of a family or "group" of schizophrenias.

Decades of research have also documented an extensive range of neuropathology in schizophrenia, including neuropsychological and cognitive deficits, neurophysiologic deficits, anatomic and functional brain abnormalities, dysfunction within several neurotransmitter systems, and a range of sleep abnormalities. This abundance of neuropathologic findings underlies the effort to identify candidate endophenotypes within the family of schizophrenias.

SLEEP CHARACTERIZATION
Subjective Assessment

In their subjective assessment of sleep, schizophrenics almost uniformly claim poor sleep quality and significant sleep disruption. Poor sleep quality may include general restlessness and agitation in addition to disturbing hypnagogic hallucinations and nightmares. Schizophrenics may also experience sleep reversals whereby the major sleep period occurs during the day with wakefulness at night. More typically, schizophrenics describe severe insomnia, particularly during episodes of relapse or the experience of positive symptoms. It is not unusual for prolonged periods of total sleeplessness to accompany states of psychotic agitation. In fact, severe insomnia is one of the prodromal signs of impending psychotic decompensation or relapse.[5] However, even with the amelioration of psychotic agitation, sleep is often characterized by a marked insomnia including long sleep-onset latency (SL), reduced total sleep time (TST), and sleep fragmented or interrupted by intervals of wakefulness. In addition, patients with schizophrenia who are medicated and clinically stable also report sleep disturbance, particularly early and middle insomnia.[6] It is also noteworthy that comorbid alcohol and substance abuse, which for some patients may reflect an attempt to self-medicate, can influence sleep quality and lead to relapse.

Objective Assessment

Many of these subjective attributes have been validated by overnight, in-laboratory, polysomnographic (PSG) studies.
Quantified PSG variables include:

- Measures of sleep maintenance, typically including:
  - SL (or the interval between "lights out" and a measure of persistent sleep)
  - TST
  - Sleep efficiency (SE), the ratio of TST to time spent in bed
- Characterization of sleep staging
  - Measures of sleep staging encompass the lighter stages N1 and N2; N3 is the deeper stage associated with slow-frequency (0–3 Hz), high-amplitude brain wave activity. Stage N3 is also referred to as slow-wave sleep (SWS). Sleep staging also includes rapid eye movement (REM) sleep time and quantification of REM sleep eye movements. The latency to the onset of the first REM period (RL) has also been the focus of many PSG studies.
- Sleep-related brain wave activity
  - Quantification of sleep-related brain activity includes slow-wave activity (SWA) in the delta band (0–3 Hz), sleep-spindle (12–15 Hz) events, and high-frequency activity (HFA) in the beta and gamma ranges (20–45 Hz).

A synopsis of PSG findings from meta-analyses and reviews is presented in **Table 1**.[7–9] These PSG studies do not always concur. Discrepancies among the findings include several sources: inclusion of diverse phenotypes, differences in protocol

Table 1 Abnormalities of sleep in schizophrenia	
Subjective Assessment	**Objective (PSG) Assessment**
Poor sleep quality	Poor sleep efficiency
Early insomnia (long sleep latency)	Reduced total sleep time
Middle insomnia	Early, middle, and late insomnia
General sleeplessness	Slow-wave sleep deficits[a]
Restlessness and agitation	Shortened REM sleep latency[a]
Sleep-wake reversals	Reduced 0–3 Hz power in non-REM sleep
Hypnagogic hallucinations	Increased 20–35 Hz and 35–45 Hz power
Nightmares	Reduced non-REM sleep spindles

Abbreviations: PSG, polysomnography; REM, rapid eye movement.
[a] Both slow-wave sleep deficits and shortened REM sleep latency are strongly represented in subgroups of patients with schizophrenia.

design, composition of control groups, sample size (statistical power), inclusion criteria (eg, age, gender, medication status and history, clinical features, and clinical history), and differences in the quantification of sleep variables.

The most consistent PSG-demonstrated sleep abnormality in schizophrenia is poor sleep maintenance, which entails a reduction in TST and increased wake time, particularly sleep-onset insomnia or difficulty reaching a state of persistent sleep. Moreover, many of these PSG studies have included patients on stable antipsychotic (AP) medication; consequently, residual insomnia can be an outcome for some AP-treated schizophrenics.

SWS deficits have been reported in about half of all PSG studies of schizophrenic patients including first-episode, AP-naïve patients.[10] Such deficits raise questions about the integrity of homeostatic regulatory mechanisms in schizophrenia. According to the homeostatic model of SWS, the homeostatic drive builds up during waking and dissipates in SWS across successive non-REM cycles.[11] In healthy subjects, SWS increases in proportion to the amount and intensity of prior waking, suggesting that this homeostatic or dynamic response serves a restorative role in brain function; in healthy controls, this dynamic response is clearly demonstrated by a rebound in SWS following the naturalistic probe of total sleep deprivation. Significantly, sleep deprivation studies in schizophrenics have found that the homeostatic drive is notably diminished.[12] Impaired or diminished restorative brain function(s) could adversely affect both clinical presentation and outcome. SWS deficits strongly characterize subgroups of schizophrenic patients, and could define an important endophenotype in the family of schizophrenias. It has been suggested that SWS deficits are a consequence of defective synaptic pruning during the second decade of life,[13] resulting in microstructural brain abnormalities.

Many PSG studies have quantified the latency to the onset of the RL, and about half have found that subgroups of schizophrenic patients have an abnormal shortening of the interval between sleep onset and the first RL. Short RL could represent a primary alteration of REM sleep mechanisms; alternatively, an SWS deficit in the first non-REM period could permit the passive advance or early onset of the RL.

Historically, the early PSG studies of sleep in schizophrenia tested the hypothesis that the pathology of schizophrenia represented, in part, the intrusion of REM sleep processes into waking. This hypothesis was never confirmed, and REM sleep is neither significantly increased nor reduced in schizophrenia. The cross-sectional study of phasic REM sleep eye movements in schizophrenics has also revealed no systematic augmentation or reduction relative to healthy controls or patients with depressive disorder.

Computer quantifications of brain-wave activity during sleep have revealed several sleep-related abnormalities. Many schizophrenics demonstrate reduced SWA relative to healthy controls, a finding broadly consistent with visually scored SWS deficits. Furthermore, HFA in the beta and gamma ranges is greater in unmedicated schizophrenics than in healthy controls, and is correlated with measures of positive symptoms. Finally, the number and amplitude of non-REM sleep spindles is less in medicated schizophrenics, a finding that would be consistent with some abnormality in thalamic-reticular and thalamocortical function in schizophrenia.

CLINICAL CORRELATES

The relationship between PSG-defined sleep variables and clinical presentation, neurocognitive impairment, and outcome has been reviewed.[14] Significant findings are shown in **Table 2**. Global symptom severity is associated with greater wake time, less SWS or stage N3, and shorter RL. Positive symptoms such as hallucinations and delusions are associated with poor SE, longer SL, shorter RL, increased REM sleep eye movement activity, and increased HFA in the underlying electroencephalogram (EEG). By contrast, negative symptoms have been related to shorter RL, SWS deficits, and their underlying delta-band SWA. Format thought disorder or cognitive dysfunction has also been associated with SWS deficits. Moreover, SWS deficits and shorter RL might predict poor clinical outcome. On tasks of neuropsychological performance, schizophrenics

Table 2
Relationship between clinical measures and sleep variables in patients with schizophrenia

Global clinical severity	Increased WAKE time; decreased SWS, RL
Positive symptoms	Increased SL, EMs, HFA; decreased SE, RL
Negative symptoms	Decreased SWS, RL, SWA
Thought disorder	Decreased SWS
Poor outcome	Decreased SWS, RL

Abbreviations: EMs, REM sleep eye movement activity; HFA, electroencephalographic (EEG) high-frequency activity; RL, REM sleep latency; SE, sleep efficiency; SL, sleep-onset latency; SWA, EEG slow-wave activity; SWS, slow-wave sleep or stage N3; WAKE, wake time after sleep onset.

with more SWS and greater delta power demonstrate better scores in measures of attention and visuospatial memory. In conclusion, these studies of clinical correlation were snapshots of clinical state or performance; longitudinal, within-patient protocols offer a better strategy with which to explore the association of changing clinical state with corresponding changes in sleep patterns.

ANTIPSYCHOTIC MEDICATION

Most patients diagnosed with schizophrenia are treated with one or more of the AP agents shown in **Table 3**. These APs have differential effects on many neurotransmitter systems including dopamine (DA), serotonin (5-HT), α-adrenergic, cholinergic, and histamine receptors.[15] Clinical outcome and the associated side effects on these APs reflect their differential receptor-binding profiles.

The first-generation APs (FGAs) were introduced in the 1950s with the release of chlorpromazine. This agent and subsequent FGAs share a common receptor profile: a high affinity for binding to the DA D_2 postsynaptic receptor. This FGA receptor-binding profile is associated not only with their efficacy in treating positive symptoms but with a range of side effects such as akathisia, dystonia, parkinsonism, tardive dyskinesia (TD), and the more lethal neuroleptic malignant syndrome. These DA-related side effects, and cholinergic side effects, are often associated with treatment noncompliance.

The impetus for the development of second-generation APs (SGAs) came from several sources: (1) many schizophrenics had an inadequate response to FGAs; (2) FGAs were not very successful in treating negative symptoms; and (3) FGA-related side effects were often associated with noncompliance and were a difficult challenge for treating clinicians. Clozapine, the first of the SGAs, was released in 1989; since then 9 additional SGAs have received approval from the Food and Drug Administration. Relative to the FGAs, the SGAs affect a broader spectrum of neurotransmitter systems; they also have a weaker affinity for the DA D_2 receptor and a stronger affinity for 5-HT receptors, particularly the 5-HT$_{2a}$ receptor. The broader receptor profile of the SGAs is associated with its own set of adverse side effects, namely, agranulocytosis, weight gain, dyslipidemias, and impaired glucose regulation. Finally, relative to the FGAs, the SGAs have a reduced incidence of extrapyramidal side effects and TD; however, EPS and TD may occur with higher doses of SGAs. Of importance is that treatment outcome and adverse side effects vary from patient to patient given the same AP regimen, and this diversity of response is consistent with the diversity of phenotypes within the family of schizophrenias.

EFFECTS OF ANTIPSYCHOTICS ON SLEEP

Broadly speaking, AP agents ameliorate the dyssomnias associated with schizophrenia. **Table 4** summarizes the results of PSG studies that evaluated AP effects on sleep.[9,15] In most instances, these studies had certain limitations. Double-blind placebo-controlled studies were rare, and many were cross-sectional comparisons that failed to use subjects as their own controls. Quetiapine and ziprasidone have been evaluated only in nonpsychiatric controls and, as yet, PSG studies of the newer SGAs (aripiprazole, asenapine, lurasidone, and iloperidone) have not been published. Despite these qualifications, both FGAs and

---

Table 3
First-generation (FGAs) and second-generation (SGAs) antipsychotic medications and range of adult daily maintenance dose

FGAs	Maintenance Dose Range (mg)	SGAs	Maintenance Dose Range (mg)
Chlorpromazine (Thorazine)	50–400	Aripiprazole (Abilify)	10–30
Fluphenazine (Prolixin)	1–15	Asenapine (Saphris)	10–20 (sublingual)
Haloperidol (Haldol)	1–15	Clozapine (Clozaril)	200–600
Perphenazine (Trilafon)	8–24	Iloperidone (Fanapt)	12–24
Thioridazine (Mellaril)	50–400	Lurasidone (Latuda)	40–160
Thiothixene (Narvane)	6–30	Olanzapine (Zyprexa)	5–20
Trifluoperazine (Stelazine)	4–30	Paliperidone (Invega)	6–12
		Quetiapine (Seroquel)	150–750
		Risperidone (Risperdal)	2–8
		Ziprasidone (Geodon)	80–160

Table 4
Effect of first-generation and second-generation antipsychotics on major PSG sleep variables

FGAs	
Chlorpromazine	Increased TST, SWS, RL; decreased SL, WASO
Thiothixene or haloperidol	Increased TST, SE, SWS, RL; decreased SL, WASO
Flupentixol or haloperidol	Increased TST, SE, stage N1; decreased SL
Haloperidol	Increased TST, stage N1, RL; decreased SL, Stage N2, decreased WASO
SGAs	
Clozapine	Increased TST, SE, stage N2; decreased SL, WASO, SWS
Olanzapine	Increased TST, SE, stage N2, SWS, TRL; decreased WASO, stage N1
Paliperidone	Increased TST, SE, stage N2; decreased SL, #WK, stage N1
Quetiapine[a]	Increased TST, SE, stage N2; decreased SL, WASO
Risperidone[b]	Increased SWS
Ziprasidone[a]	Increased TST, SE, stage N2, SWS, RL; decreased WASO, #WK, stage N1

Abbreviations: FGAs, first-generation antipsychotics; N1, non-REM Stage 1; N2, non-REM stage 2; RL, REM latency; SE, sleep efficiency; SGAs, second-generation antipsychotics; SL, sleep-onset latency; SWS, slow-wave sleep or stage N3; TST, total sleep time; WASO, waking minutes after sleep onset; #WK, number of awakenings.
[a] Studied only nonpsychiatric controls.
[b] Risperidone relative only to haloperidol.

SGAs seem to improve both sleep maintenance and sleep architecture in many schizophrenic patients. All APs tested on schizophrenic patients documented some sedating effects, either decreasing SL and wake time or increasing TST or SE. With the notable exception of clozapine, SWS augmentation was observed in PSG studies of certain FGAs (ie, chlorpromazine and thiothixene) and SGAs (ie, olanzapine and risperidone, and ziprasidone). In the risperidone study, the SWS enhancement was relative to SWS amounts observed with haloperidol. As a final point, monotherapy with an SGA is standard practice; however, therapeutic response may be optimized with an additional AP. Also, it is not uncommon for other psychoactive medications to be prescribed for comorbid psychiatric illness; for example, antidepressants and mood stabilizers. These agents may also have a beneficial effect on the dyssomnias of schizophrenia.

COMORBID SLEEP DISORDERS IN ANTIPSYCHOTIC-TREATED SCHIZOPHRENICS
Insomnia

Despite treatment with AP agents, it is not uncommon for schizophrenics to complain of unresolved insomnia. In fact, rates of residual insomnia in AP-treated schizophrenics range from 16% to 30%.[16] Often this insomnia can be attributed to inadequate or undertreated hyperarousal or to sleep-related movement disorders.

As reviewed earlier, insomnia is the most consistently reported dyssomnia associated with schizophrenia. Long SL and poor SE are emblematic of the hyperarousal and psychotic turmoil associated with schizophrenia. Because AP agents are associated with a range of potentially adverse side effects, clinicians typically prescribe the lowest maintenance dose with clinical efficacy. Consequently, some degree of hyperarousal and residual insomnia may characterize a subset of schizophrenics on maintenance doses of APs. Treating this comorbid insomnia may require: (1) increasing the dose of the prescribed AP agent; (2) switching medications to a more sedating AP; or (3) adding a low dose of a more sedating AP. Among the currently approved AP agents, chlorpromazine, thioridazine, clozapine, olanzapine, risperidone, and iloperidone provide relatively more sedation. Another approach clinicians might consider is the adjunctive use of an anxiolytic or sedative hypnotic; however, such medications should be prescribed cautiously, particularly for schizophrenics with sleep-related breathing disorders (SBDs) or a history of alcohol or drug abuse.

Other sources of insomnia in AP-treated schizophrenics are sleep-related movement disorders such as restless legs syndrome (RLS) and periodic limb movement disorder (PLMD). Baseline prevalence rates for these disorders in AP-naïve schizophrenics have never been established. However, because RLS and PLMD respond favorably to DA agonists, a DA deficiency is a likely component of their pathophysiology.[17] As a consequence, AP agents, with their D_2 receptor blockade, might contribute to or induce RLS or PLMD as an adverse side effect. Indeed, prevalence rates of RLS in AP-treated schizophrenics are reported to be more than twice that of healthy controls.[18] RLS and PLMD have been documented in patients taking SGAs such as riperidone,[19] olanzapine,[20,21] quetiapine,[22] and clozapine.[23] Not all AP-treated schizophrenics develop RLS; therefore, it has been suggested that a necessary precondition lies in a genetic risk factor such as a polymorphism of the *BTBD9* gene.[24]

Like the diagnosis of schizophrenia, RLS is a clinical diagnosis meeting certain criteria.[25] RLS is associated with significant sleep-onset insomnia and more severe psychiatric symptoms. By contrast, the diagnosis of PLMD requires a PSG recording of leg-movement activity and associated EEG arousals. PLMD is associated with complaints of restless or unrefreshing sleep. Patients with RLS typically also present with PLMD. For schizophrenics with RLS or PLMD, standard treatment with DA agonists such as ropinirole, pramipexole, or rotigotine is not recommended. Instead, clinicians might switch to a different AP agent; alternatively gabapentin or pregabalin may be added to the ongoing AP regimen. Possible iron deficiency should also be assessed, as this is now known to be a risk factor for the development of RLS.[26] Finally, clinicians are often faced with the task of differentiating comorbid RLS from AP-induced akathisia. Although RLS has a more marked circadian component (with greater severity in the evening), the distinction can at times prove difficult. Akathisia is also a source of sleep disruption, and may be treated with propranolol or benztropine.

Hypersomnia

In contrast to insomnia in AP-treated schizophrenics, rates of hypersomnia suggest a more pervasive problem. Between 24% and 31% of AP-treated schizophrenics report daytime somnolence.[16] This level of somnolence may be a direct adverse effect of some AP agents or symptomatic of an SBD enhanced by or induced by AP medication.

Among the FGAs, somnolence is associated with the high-milligram, low-potency agents such as chlorpromazine and thioridazine. Clozapine is well recognized as the most sedating of the SGAs. Risperidone and olanzapine, though not as sedating as clozapine, are known for increased somnolence. Although somnolence may be associated with certain APs, sleepiness is also affected by the half-life of the AP, amount of drug, and dosing schedule. Because daytime somnolence may impair function and decrease the quality of life, somnolence secondary to AP treatment is usually addressed by changing AP medication or reducing dosage. Recent case studies determined that aripiprazole improved both psychotic symptoms and daytime somnolence when added to ongoing clozapine therapy.[27]

SBDs such as obstructive sleep apnea (OSA) may be another source of somnolence in AP-treated schizophrenics. In a study of schizophrenic patients referred to a sleep clinic for a suspected sleep disorder, more than 46% met criteria for OSA, with obesity being the best predictor.[28] Because weight gain is a frequent adverse side effect of many APs, OSA may be exacerbated or induced by these agents. Weight gain as a side effect of AP treatment has been associated with the use of both FGAs and SGAs such as chlorpromazine, thioridazine, clozapine, olanzapine, and risperidone. Morbid obesity and the development of moderate to severe SDB have been observed in both clozapine and risperidone treatment.[29] It is interesting that significant weight loss was observed when aripiprazole was substituted for, or added as an adjunct to, olanzapine.[30,31] Finally, the diagnosis of comorbid OSA must be considered for those schizophrenics who are somnolent and historically obese, or who have gained weight during the course of AP treatment. These patients can be treated successfully with continuous positive airway pressure, and demonstrate both good compliance and significant clinical improvement.[32]

Parasomnias

Parasomnias occur against a backdrop of a partial arousal from SWS. Schizophrenics may be at risk of developing a parasomnia if they are prescribed a psychotropic agent known to increase SWS. Examples of parasomnias include sleepwalking (somnambulism) and sleep-related eating disorders, both of which have been associated with AP treatment. Somnambulism has been observed when lithium has been added to FGAs[33] or following treatment with olanzapine.[34] Finally, sleep-related eating disorders have been linked to APs such as olanzapine and risperidone.[35,36]

REFERENCES

1. McGrath J, Saha S, Chant D, et al. Schizophrenia: a concise overview of incidence, prevalence, and mortality. Epidemiol Rev 2008;30:67–76.
2. American Psychiatric Association. Diagnostic and statistical manual of mental disorders. 5th edition. Arlington (VA): American Psychiatric Press; 2013.
3. Sullivan PF, Kendler KS, Neale MC. Schizophrenia as a complex trait. Arch Gen Psychiatry 2003;60: 1187–92.
4. Svrakic DM, Zorumski CF, Svrakic NM, et al. Risk architecture of schizophrenia: the role of epigenetics. Curr Opin Psychiatry 2013;26:188–95.
5. Chemerinski E, Ho B, Flaum M, et al. Insomnia as a predictor for symptom worsening following antipsychotic withdrawal in schizophrenia. Compr Psychiatry 2002;43:393–6.

6. Haffmans PM, Hoencamp E, Knegtering HJ, et al. Sleep disturbance in schizophrenia. Br J Psychiatry 1994;165:697–8.
7. Benca RM, Obermeyer WH, Thisted RA, et al. Sleep and psychiatric disorders: a meta-analysis. Arch Gen Psychiatry 1992;49:651–68.
8. Chouinard S, Poulin J, Stip E, et al. Sleep in un-treated patients with schizophrenia: a meta-analysis. Schizophr Bull 2004;30(4):957–67.
9. Benson KL, Feinberg I. Schizophrenia. In: Kryger MH, Roth T, Dement WC, editors. Principles and practice of sleep medicine. 5th edition. Philadelphia: Elsevier Saunders; 2010. p. 1501–11.
10. Poulin J, Daoust A, Forest G, et al. Sleep architecture and its clinical correlates in first episode and neuroleptic-naive patients with schizophrenia. Schizophr Res 2003;62:147–53.
11. Feinberg I. Changes in sleep cycle patterns with age. J Psychiatr Res 1974;10:283–306.
12. Luby ED, Caldwell DF. Sleep deprivation and EEG slow wave activity in chronic schizophrenia. Arch Gen Psychiatry 1967;17:361–4.
13. Feinberg I. Schizophrenia: caused by a fault in programmed synaptic elimination during adolescence? J Psychiatr Res 1983;17:319–34.
14. Benson KL. Sleep in schizophrenia. Sleep Med Clin 2008;3:251–60.
15. Krystal AD, Goforth HW, Roth T. Effects of antipsychotic medications on sleep in schizophrenia. Int Clin Psychopharmacol 2008;23:150–60.
16. Lieberman JA, Stroup TS, McEvoy JP, et al. Effectiveness of antipsychotic drugs in patients with chronic schizophrenia. N Engl J Med 2005;353(12):1209–23.
17. Allen RP, Earley CJ. Restless legs syndrome: a review of clinical and pathophysiologic features. J Clin Neurophysiol 2001;18:128–47.
18. Kang SG, Lee HJ, Jung SW, et al. Characteristics and clinical correlates of restless legs syndrome in schizophrenia. Pharmacopsychiatry 2007;31:1078–83.
19. Wetter TC, Brunner J, Bronisch T. Restless legs syndrome probably induced by risperidone treatment. Pharmacopsychiatry 2002;35:109–11.
20. Khalid I, Rana L, Khalid TJ, et al. Refractory restless legs syndrome likely caused by olanzapine. J Clin Sleep Med 2009;5:68–9.
21. Kang SG, Lee HJ, Kim L. Restless legs syndrome and periodic limb movements during sleep probably associated with olanzapine. J Psychopharmacol 2009;23:597–601.
22. Pinninti NR, Mago R, Townsend J, et al. Periodic restless legs syndrome associated with quetiapine. J Clin Psychopharmacol 2005;25:617–8.
23. Duggal HS, Mendhekar DN. Clozapine-associated restless les syndrome. J Clin Psychopharmacol 2007;27:89–90.
24. Kang SG, Lee HJ, Park YM, et al. The BTBD9 gene may be associated with antipsychotic-induced restless legs syndrome in schizophrenia. Hum Psychopharmacol 2013;28:117–23.
25. Allen R, Henning W, Montplaisir J, et al. Restless legs syndrome: diagnostic criteria, special considerations, and epidemiology: a report from the RLS Diagnosis and Epidemiology Workshop at the National Institutes of Health. Sleep Med 2003;4:101–19.
26. Allen R. Dopamine and iron in the pathophysiology of restless legs syndrome (RLS). Sleep Med 2004;5:385–91.
27. Rocha FL, Hara C. Benefits of combining aripiprazole to clozapine: three case reports. Prog Neuropsychopharmacol Biol Psychiatry 2006;30:1167–9.
28. Winkelman JW. Schizophrenia, obesity, and obstructive sleep apnea. J Clin Psychiatry 2001;62:8–11.
29. Wirshing DA, Pierre JM, Wirshing WC. Sleep apnea associated with antipsychotic-induced obesity. J Clin Psychiatry 2002;63:369–70.
30. Newcomer JW, Campos JA, Marcus RN, et al. A multicenter, randomized, double-blind study of the effects of aripiprazole in overweight subjects with schizophrenia or schizoaffective disorder switched from olanzapine. J Clin Psychiatry 2008;69:1046–56.
31. Henderson DC, Fan X, Copeland PM. Aripiprazole added to overweight and obese olanzapine-treated schizophrenic patients. J Clin Psychopharmacol 2009;29:165–9.
32. Karanti A, Landén M. Treatment refractory psychosis remitted upon treatment with continuous positive airway pressure: a case report. Psychopharmacol Bull 2007;40:113–7.
33. Charney DS, Kales A, Soldatos CR, et al. Somnambulistic-like episodes secondary to combined lithium-neuroleptic treatment. Br J Psychiatry 1979;135:418–24.
34. Kolivakis TT, Margolese HC, Beauclair L, et al. Olanzapine-induced somnambulism. Am J Psychiatry 2001;158:1158.
35. Paquet V, Strul J, Servais L, et al. Sleep-related eating disorder induced by olanzapine. J Clin Psychiatry 2002;63:597.
36. Lu ML, Shen WW. Sleep-related eating disorder induced by risperidone. J Clin Psychiatry 2004;65:273.

Non–Benzodiazepine Receptor Agonists for Insomnia

Philip M. Becker, MD[a,b,*], Manya Somiah, MD[b]

KEYWORDS

- Non–benzodiazepine receptor agonists • BZRA • Insomnia • Z-drugs

KEY POINTS

- Benzodiazepines receptor agonists such as zolpidem, zaleplon, and eszopiclone show favorable efficacy and safety in double-blind, placebo-controlled trials for transient and chronic insomnia whether of primary and comorbid origin.
- Management of chronic insomnia requires assessment for underlying causes through comprehensive assessment of biological, psychological, and lifestyle factors.
- Because onset of action is similar among the agents, half-life differentiates 1 Z-drug from another.
- Zolpidem controlled release or eszopiclone have different binding characteristics of receptor subtypes and likely have some differences that do not make them equivalent hypnotic agents.
- For the foreseeable future, the Z-drugs will continue to be the principal pharmaceuticals to improve chronic insomnia.

The pharmacologic management of insomnia, whether acute or chronic, commonly includes the use of agents that are active at the benzodiazepine–γ-aminobutyric acid (GABA) complex, particularly receptors in the ventrolateral preoptic (VLPO) nucleus. Because of proven efficacy, reduced side effects, and lesser concern about addiction, non–benzodiazepine receptor agonists (non-BzRAs) have become the most commonly prescribed hypnotic agents that are approved to treat onset and maintenance insomnia. Non-BzRAs are frequently referred to as the Z-drugs, because the approved sedative/hypnotic agents in the United States include zaleplon, zolpidem, and eszopiclone (a derivative of zopiclone). In a review of the clinical evaluation and management of chronic insomnia,[1] practice guidelines of the American Academy of Sleep Medicine provided a consensus opinion that first-line treatment is cognitive-behavioral therapy. When

pharmacologic treatment is indicated, non-BzRAs are first-line agents for the short-term and long-term management of transient and chronic insomnia related to adjustment, psychophysiologic, primary, and secondary causation. In this article, the benefits and risks of non-BzRAs and the selection of a hypnotic agent is defined, based on efficacy, pharmacologic profile, and adverse events.

A BRIEF REVIEW OF SEDATIVE-HYPNOTIC AGENTS

Alcohol, a central nervous system (CNS) depressant that interacts with GABA receptors, has been the most used agent for problems of sleep throughout human history, although it disturbs sleep in the last half of the night.[2] Chloral hydrate is a CNS depressant that acts rapidly through its reduced metabolite, trichloroethanol, and the $GABA_A$

[a] Department of Psychiatry, University of Texas Southwestern Medical Center at Dallas, Dallas, TX, USA;
[b] Sleep Medicine Associates of Texas, 5477 Glen Lakes Drive, Suite 100, Dallas, TX 75231, USA
* Corresponding author. Sleep Medicine Associates of Texas, 5477 Glen Lakes Drive, Suite 100, Dallas, TX 75231.
E-mail address: pbecker@sleepmed.com

Sleep Med Clin 10 (2015) 57–76
http://dx.doi.org/10.1016/j.jsmc.2014.11.002
1556-407X/15/$ – see front matter © 2015 Elsevier Inc. All rights reserved.

receptor system.[3] Bromides are broad CNS depressants that have an uncertain mechanism of action.[4] There are multiple barbituric acid derivatives such as phenobarbital, amobarbital, pentobarbital, and secobarbital, as well as barbituratelike compounds (ethchlorvinyl, meprobamate, methyprylon, glutethimide). As doses increase, barbiturates carry risks for addiction and side effects, including accidental overdose or suicide. Barbiturates inhibit the closure of the GABA$_A$ chloride channel, altering the rate of chloride diffusion and resulting action potentials.[5] Benzodiazepines proved a significant advance, because they proved safer and of better longer-term benefit in the management of chronic insomnia. Because benzodiazepines occupy GABA$_A$ receptors throughout the brain, side effects, including balance, memory, and addiction potential, became potentially problematic. More receptor-specific non-BzRAs proved an advance as the understanding of neural networks/anatomy of sleep regulation expanded.

PHARMACOLOGY OF γ-AMINOBUTYRIC ACID A COMPLEX

GABA is the main inhibitory neurotransmitter in the mammalian CNS. GABA$_A$ receptors consist of 19 pentameric protein subunits from 7 distinct gene families (α, β, γ, δ, ε, θ, and π). The sites of non-BzRA action typically contain α$_1$, α$_2$, α$_3$, or α$_5$, β$_2$ or β$_3$, and γ$_2$ subunits.[6] Non-BzRAs are chemically distinct from benzodiazepines and bind selectively to the GABA$_A$ receptors, the proposed action that improves sleep.

ZOLPIDEM

Zolpidem is an imidazopyridine[7] that increases the affinity of GABA to GABA$_A$ receptors and results in inhibition through longer opening of the chloride channel, which increases cell membrane potential.[8] Zolpidem is available in tablet, sublingual, and oral spray mist formulations. Zolpidem at hypnotic dosages binds selectively to the α$_1$ subunit of the GABA$_A$ complex.[9,10] It binds with a 10-fold lower affinity to α$_2$ and α$_3$ receptor subtypes, which are associated with anxiolysis and enhanced mood in animal models.[11,12] Zolpidem shows no appreciable affinity for α$_5$ subunit receptors. The primary locations of α$_1$ subtype receptors are on lamina IV of the sensorimotor cortex, pars reticulata, cerebellum, olfactory bulb, ventrolateral preoptic complex of thalamus, inferior colliculus, and globus pallidus.[13]

Pharmacology

Zolpidem is rapidly absorbed after oral administration and undergoes first-pass metabolism. It has a short half-life (2.2 hours), attaining peak plasma concentration in 1.5 to 2.5 hours. Standard adult doses are available as immediate release (IR) at 5 mg and 10 mg and controlled release (CR) at 6.25 mg and 12.5 mg[14] and a new middle of the night (MOTN) dosing of 1.75 mg for women and 3.5 mg for men. Zolpidem is principally metabolized by hepatic cytochrome enzymes.[15,16] Induction or inhibition of these enzymes by other drugs can alter plasma levels of zolpidem. **Table 1** provides a detailed description of the pharmacology of zolpidem.

Indications/Uses

Tables 2 and **3** describe the pivotal trials that supported the approval of zolpidem for transient and chronic insomnia. Standard IR formulations of zolpidem 5 and 10 mg are approved for short-term treatment of sleep onset insomnia.[17,18] IR preparations shorten sleep latency and improve next day functioning.[19–22] CR preparations are approved for sleep onset and sleep maintenance insomnia.[23–25] Study of IR 7.5 mg and 10 mg showed significant improvement in a model of transient insomnia that involved circadian misalignment to produce the insomnia by advancing bedtime by 4 hours from the patient's routine.[26] Persistent insomnia in depressed individuals who are treated with selective serotonin reuptake inhibitors (SSRIs) improves with concurrent zolpidem.[27] Zolpidem IR is used to improve sleep and mission readiness in pilots,[28] and it also improves altitude insomnia in mountain climbers without affecting respiration, attention, alertness, or mood.[29] As needed use rather than nightly zolpidem has been recommended, and several studies support use up to 3 nights per week. Intermittent use during a week is both effective and well tolerated, with little tendency to increase hypnotic intake over time.[30,31] All forms of nightly or as needed use of zolpidem should be taken immediately before bedtime to reduce confusional episodes in or around sleep. The US Food and Drug Administration (FDA) has approved a sublingual form of zolpidem to treat insomnia characterized by MOTN waking, with difficulty returning to sleep. Doses differ by gender, at 1.75 mg for women and 3.5 mg for men. Zolpidem should be taken only if at least 4 hours of bedtime remain before final awakening for the day. This is the lowest dose formulation of zolpidem available commercially.[32]

Cautions

At doses of 20 to 200 mg, zolpidem binds to all benzodiazepine receptors, producing both

Table 1
Pharmacology of zolpidem, zaleplon, and eszopiclone

	Zolpidem	Zaleplon	Eszopiclone[a,145,180–182]
Half-life (h)	IR and CR: adults 2.2[81,183] IR: children ≈1.4[9] IR and CR: Elderly ≈2.8[184,185] IR and CR: hepatic insufficiency ≈9.9[9]	1[186,187]	Adults: 6 Elderly: 9[188]
Peak plasma concentration (h)	IR and CR: 1.5–2.5	1[186,187]	1
Absorption	IR and CR: rapid oral	Rapid oral[124,186]	Rapid oral
Bioavailability (%)	IR and CR: 70[9,189]	30[124,186]	80 (racemic zopiclone)
Plasma protein binding (%)	IR and CR: 92[9,189]	60 (lipophilic)	52–59
Factors interfering with absorption	IR and CR: large meals	Large, fatty meals	Large, fatty meals
C_{max}	IR (5 mg and 10 mg): 59 ng/mL and 121 ng/mL CR (12.5 mg): 134 ng/mL	10 mg–37 ng/mL	87.3 ng/mL
Kinetics	IR and CR: linear[14]	Linear[186]	Linear
Metabolism	IR and CR: CYP3A4 (major) CYP1A2 (minor)	Aldehyde oxidase (major) CYP3A4 (minor)	Oxidation, demethylation[190] CYP3A4, CYP2E1,[123] CYP2C8[191] in vitro
Drug interactions (concentration)	Inducers of CYP system[b] (decrease) Inhibitors of CYP system[c] (increase)[192]	Inhibitors of CYP system[c] (increase, 30%)[94,193] Inducers of CYP system[b] and aldehyde oxidase[d] (decrease, 80%)	Inducers of CYP system[b] (decrease) Inhibitors of CYP system[c] (increase)
Activity of metabolites	IR and CR: inactive	Inactive	(S)-zopiclone-N-oxide: inactive (S)-N-desmethyl zopiclone: active
Modes of excretion (%)	IR and CR: renal (96)[14]	Renal (71) Gastrointestinal (17)	Renal (75) 10 unchanged drug in urine
Adjusted dose requirements	Elderly Children Hepatic impairment CNS-active drugs	Hepatic impairment: mild/ moderate/severe Renal impairment: severe CNS-active drugs: ethanol/ imipramine/thioridazine (reversed within 1–4 h of administration)[194]	Elderly Hepatic impairment: severe

Abbreviation: C_{max}, peak serum concentration that a drug achieves after single administration.
[a] Single doses of ≤7.5 mg and once-daily administration of 1.0, 3.0, and 6.0 mg for 7 days.
[b] Inducers: anticonvulsants: carbamazepine, phenytoin; barbiturates: phenobarbital; bactericidals; rifampicin, rifabutin; nonnucleoside reverse transcriptase inhibitors: efavirenz, nevirapine; hypoglycemics: pioglitazone; glucocorticoids: modafinil.
[c] Inhibitors: macrolides: clarithromycin; azole antifungals: ketoconazole, itraconazole/chloramphenicol/nefazodone; protease inhibitors: ritonavir, indinavir/cimetidine.
[d] Cimetidine.

anticonvulsant and muscle-relaxant effects.[33] Use in pregnancy is classified under category C. Animal studies have shown adverse fetal effects of decreased skull ossification at 24 to 120 times the recommended human dose.[34,35] Wikner and Källén[36] reported no increase in fetal malformation risks from zolpidem IR 5 to 10 mg during pregnancy. Wang and colleagues[37] reported low birth

Table 2
Zolpidem use in transient insomnia

	Roth et al,[26] 1995
Study design	Placebo-controlled double-blind parallel group study with unbalanced randomization during experimental phase advance
Number of patients	462 normal volunteers
Entry criteria	Transient insomnia (first night effect by phase advance) (Koshorek et al,[195]; Monti et al,[196] 1993)
Number of drug evaluation nights	Single night
Dosage (mg)	Placebo; zolpidem 5, 7.5, 10, 15, 20 Statistical analysis of 7.5, 10 zolpidem was compared with placebo
Assessment of sleep	Polysomnography
Subjective results	Zolpidem 7.5 mg • Mean sleep latency: decreased ($P = .009$) Zolpidem 10 mg • Mean sleep latency: decreased ($P<.001$)
Objective results	Zolpidem 7.5 mg • Mean sleep latency: decreased ($P<.001$) • Sleep efficiency: increased ($P<.001$) • Number of awakenings: decreased ($P = .004$) • Wake time during sleep: decreased ($P = .004$) Zolpidem 10 mg • Mean sleep latency: decreased ($P<.001$) • Sleep efficiency: increased ($P<.001$) • Number of awakenings: decreased ($P = .014$) • Wake time during sleep: decreased ($P = .005$)
Conclusion	• Zolpidem at 7.5 mg and 10 mg is effective treating transient insomnia • No effect on next day psychomotor performance

weight and small for gestational age babies in a population-based study of mothers on zolpidem. A single case of fetal neural tube defects occurred in the baby of a woman who took higher than recommended doses of zolpidem during the first trimester.[38] Despite minimal excretion of zolpidem into breast milk, alternatives to zolpidem during breastfeeding should be considered.[39] The recommended doses for zolpidem in women have been reduced, as stated in a recent ruling by the FDA. The science of this recommendation is explained later.

Abuse

Zolpidem can be abused. Recreational users taking higher than therapeutic doses report vivid visuals and a high while fighting to stay awake. Abusers crave its anxiolytic and stimulating properties to help cope with everyday activities.[40] Gericke and Ludolph[41] presented a report of zolpidem being chronically abused at very high doses and described the effects of overdose. As a result of availability of liquid and sublingual forms of zolpidem, there is concern about use as a date rape drug in lieu of rohypnol.

Novel Off-Label Use

Zolpidem may improve aphasia for a short duration in patients with stroke[42] and is being investigated in patients with disorders of consciousness, such as minimally conscious state, aphasia, gait disorders, and akinetic mutism.[43–51] Snyman and colleagues[52] used zolpidem to treat pediatric patients in a persistent vegetative state and concluded that zolpidem had no beneficial effect in pediatric patients. Despite numerous case reports of improvements in alertness in patients with disorders of consciousness, definitive evidence is lacking, and a more thorough controlled investigation is needed. Garretto and colleagues[53] showed improvement in blepharospasm and Meige syndrome, postulating that zolpidem alters basal ganglia function. Wang and colleagues[54] reported transient improvements in facial expression, speech, and smooth limb movement in postsurgical central pontine myelinolysis. Zolpidem is also reported to improve behavioral and motor symptoms on discontinuation of haloperidol in schizoaffective disorder,[55] spinocerebellar ataxia,[56] postanoxic spasticity,[57] restless leg syndrome,[58] progressive supranuclear palsy[59] and in Parkinson disease and parkinsonian features.[60–63] Cerebellar mutism syndrome after posterior fossa surgery of medulloblastoma is affected by zolpidem, increasing arousal and decreasing emotional lability.[64]

Adverse Effects

Adverse events include gastrointestinal upset, headaches, disinhibition, and potential effects on most CNS functions. Anterograde amnesia and short-term memory loss are of primary concern around peak plasma level if the patient remains awake after ingestion or spontaneously wakes. These effects are dose related, occurring within 30 minutes of ingestion, but are not usually associated with serious abnormal behavior.[65–67] Up to 15% of users have no memory of events or behaviors that occur during their sleep.[67–69] Significant effects on recent and remote recall have been reported.[70] Hallucinations or sensory distortions seem more common in women at doses greater than 5 mg per day and with concomitant inhibitors of the CYP450 isoenzyme system.[71] Five percent of users have reported sleep eating,[72,73] somnambulism,[74–76] driving, and other purposeful behavior while sleeping. These events of confusional arousal may occur with high doses, rapid increases in serum concentration,[66,68] or when zolpidem is combined with CNS-active medications or alcohol.[66] A previous history of brain injury may make patients more susceptible.[77] In such affected individuals, nocturnal activity (ie, walking, eating, or driving) occurs and is subsequently not recalled after returning to sleep, possibly because of the sedation-mediated amnestic properties of zolpidem, which could affect hippocampal memory consolidation.[65] The mechanisms of the disruption of memory by zolpidem remain poorly understood and need further investigation.[78]

Some evidence of hangover effects of zolpidem after night-time administration are described, raising concerns in the elderly of increased risks of falls and next day driving performance,[79,80] leading to the recommendation for the initial dose of 5 mg or less in view of their decreased clearance.[81,82] Daytime driving simulator tests in healthy young adults after bedtime zolpidem showed comparable results against placebo in collisions and deviation from speed limit or absolute speed.[83] Combining zolpidem with alcohol and other sedative agents should be carefully considered, because of additive effects with potential performance decrements.[84,85]

Physical tolerance and dependence to zolpidem can develop during regular, extended use. Zolpidem should be gradually withdrawn over weeks to prevent a withdrawal reaction, which resembles benzodiazepine withdrawal. A long-acting benzodiazepine like diazepam or chlordiazepoxide can be used as a substitute and subsequently withdrawn gradually. An inpatient rapid detoxification program with flumazenil has been described as treatment of zolpidem addiction.[86,87] Overdose may cause excessive sedation, pinpoint pupils, and respiratory failure progressing to coma with loss of brainstem reflexes and possibly death.[88,89] Overdoses have also been treated with flumazenil.[90] Pregabalin, a newer antiepileptic with various therapeutic uses, has been reported as successful in the treatment of zolpidem abuse, dependence, and withdrawal.[91]

ZALEPLON

Zaleplon is a pyrazolopyrimidine compound with affinity for similar $GABA_A$ receptors to zolpidem.[92] Zaleplon is the shortest acting approved hypnotic agent in the United States. It resembles zolpidem in its mechanism of action and side effect profile. However, because of its shorter duration of action, zaleplon is associated with fewer residual effects. Withdrawal reactions on abrupt cessation of zaleplon are significantly less when compared with zolpidem.

Pharmacology

A comprehensive description of the pharmacology of zaleplon is provided in **Table 1**. Zaleplon is well absorbed orally but undergoes significant first-pass metabolism. The standard adult dose available is 5-mg or 10-mg capsules. Zaleplon is primarily metabolized by hepatic enzymes.[93,94] Compounds interfering with these enzymes result in a change in plasma concentrations and may require changes in dosing. Pharmacokinetics are unaffected by gender, age, or mild to moderate renal dysfunction.[95] Use in severe hepatic and renal impairment, known hypersensitivity reactions to the agent or its constituents, sleep apnea syndrome, myasthenia gravis, severe respiratory insufficiency, and children is potentially contraindicated and requires discussion of risks and close observation in the first weeks of administration.

Indications/Uses

Zaleplon is effective in promoting initiation of sleep at 5, 10, and 20 mg.[92,96,97] Its use for sleep maintenance insomnia at 5 and 20 mg, both in IR and modified release (MR) preparations, has also been investigated.[98–102] Zaleplon is indicated for the treatment of chronic primary insomnia.[99] Pivotal trials that determined the uses of zaleplon are presented in **Tables 4–6**. Because of its short

Table 3
Zolpidem use in chronic primary insomnia

	Scharf et al,[19] 1994	Perlis et al,[22] 2004	Walsh et al,[21] 2000
Study design	Randomized double-blind placebo-controlled parallel group multicenter	Randomized large-scale double-blind placebo-controlled long-term	Randomized double-blind placebo-controlled parallel groups multicenter
Number of patients	75	199	163 (134 completed study)
Entry criteria	DSM-IV criteria for primary insomnia	DSM-IV criteria for primary insomnia	DSM-IV criteria for primary insomnia
Number of drug evaluation nights	35-night treatment period	3-night posttreatment period (assess rebound)	12 wk (take medication as needed, ≥3 nights to no more than 5 nights/wk)	8 wk (take medication as needed, ≥3 nights to no more than 5 nights/wk)
Dosage (mg)	Placebo; zolpidem 10, 15	Placebo; zolpidem 10	Placebo; zolpidem 10
Assessment of sleep	Polysomnography Self-reports	Self-reports (sleep diaries with pill use recorded)	Self-reports Investigator reports
Subjective results	• Helped fall asleep	• Sleep latency: decrease (42%) • Number of awakenings: decrease (52%) • WASO: decrease (55%) • Total sleep time: increase (27%)	• PGR[a]: effective in initiating and maintaining sleep • IGR[b]: reduced insomnia severity, better therapeutic benefit • Sleep latency: decrease • Number of awakenings: decrease • Total sleep time: increase • Quality of sleep: improved • Rebound insomnia: absent

Objective results	• Sleep latency:
	  decrease
	  (10–15 mg)
	• Sleep efficiency:
	  improved
	  (10–15 mg)
	• WASO: comparable
	  with placebo
	• Stage N3 sleep:
	  preserved
	  (10–15 mg)
	• Rapid eye move-
	  ment sleep: decrease
	  in wk 3 and 4
	  (15 mg)
	• Tolerance: absent
	  (10–15 mg)
		• Sleep latency: decrease (10 mg)
		• Sleep efficiency: improved
		  (10 mg)

Conclusions	• 10 mg of zolpidem safe and effective • 15 mg zolpidem has no clinical advantage over 10 mg • No evidence of rebound insomnia	• 10 mg zolpidem significantly improved sleep continuity on intermittent use • No evidence of rebound insomnia or dose escalation	• 10 mg zolpidem effective when used intermittently • No evidence of discontinuation effects or increased frequency of pill taking

Abbreviations: DSM-IV, Diagnostic and Statistical Manual of Mental Disorders, Fourth Edition; WASO, wake after sleep onset.
[a] Patient Global Rating: 1 = marked worsening, 7 = marked improvement.
[b] Investigator Global Rating: 1 = normal, not at all ill, 7 = extremely severe.

Table 4
Zaleplon use in sleep initiation

	Elie et al,[92] 1999	Fry et al,[97] 2000
Study design	Randomized double-blind placebo-controlled and active comparator–controlled multicenter	Placebo-controlled and active comparator–controlled
Entry criteria	DSM-III-R insomnia	Outpatients with insomnia
Number of drug evaluation nights	7 nights placebo baseline 28 nights treatment 3 nights placebo	4 wk
Dosage (mg)	Placebo; zaleplon 5, 10, 20 mg; zolpidem 10 mg	Placebo; zaleplon 5, 10, 20 mg; zolpidem 10 mg
Assessment of sleep	Sleep questionnaires	Sleep questionnaires
Subjective results	Zolpidem • Sleep latency: decrease • Sleep duration: increase • Quality of sleep: improved • Rebound insomnia: present • Withdrawal: present Zaleplon • Sleep latency: decrease (10–20 mg/all weeks, 5 mg/first 3 wk) • Sleep duration: increase (20 mg/all but week 3) • Rebound insomnia: absent • Withdrawal: absent	Zolpidem • Sleep latency: decrease • Sleep duration: increase • Quality of sleep: improved • Rebound insomnia: present • Withdrawal: present Zaleplon • Sleep latency: decrease (5–20 mg/wk 1, 10 mg/wk 3, 20 mg/all weeks) • Number of awakenings: decrease (20 mg) • Sleep duration: increase (20 mg) • Quality of sleep: improved (20 mg) • Rebound insomnia: absent • Withdrawal: absent • Tolerance: absent
Conclusions	• Zaleplon effectively treats insomnia • No evidence of withdrawal or rebound insomnia • Favorable safety profile	• Zaleplon provides effective treatment of insomnia • Favorable safety profile

Abbreviation: DSM-III-R, Diagnostic and Statistical Manual of Mental Disorders, Third Edition Revised.

Table 5
Zaleplon in sleep maintenance

	Stone et al,[98] 2002	Zammit et al,[100] 2006
Study design	Randomized double-blind placebo-controlled and active drug-controlled 4-period crossover	Randomized double-blind placebo-controlled 3-period crossover
Number of patients	13 healthy volunteers	37 patients
Entry criteria	Normal hearing, who were sensitive to sleep-disrupting effects of noise	Sleep maintenance insomnia
Number of drug evaluation nights	6	3
Dosage (mg)	Placebo; zaleplon 10, 20; zopiclone 7.5	Placebo; zaleplon 10; zolpidem 10
Assessment of sleep	Sleep questionnaires Electroencephalograph Psychomotor performance and memory tests	Polysomnography Sleep latency for residual sedation Self-reports
Subjective results	Zaleplon No residual effects Zopiclone Impaired memory on: • Delayed recall of words ($P = .001$) • Attenuated DSST ($P = .004$) • Attenuated CRT ($P = .001$)	Zaleplon • No significant differences in daytime sedation measures Zolpidem • Sleep onset on latency testing: decrease (4, 5, 7 h after zolpidem; $P<.001$, $P<.001$, $P<.05$) • Concentration: decrease (4, 5, 6 h after zolpidem; $P<.05$, $P<.05$, $P<.05$) • Alertness: decrease (4 h after zolpidem; $P<.05$) • DSST: decrease (4, 5 h after zolpidem; $P<.001$, $P<.001$)
Objective results	Zaleplon • Sleep latency: decrease (10 mg, $P = .001$; 20 mg, $P = .014$) • Stage 1 sleep: decrease (20 mg, $P = .012$) Zopiclone • Stage 1 sleep: decrease ($P = .001$) • Stage 3 sleep: increase ($P = .0001$) • Total sleep time: increase ($P = .003$)	Zaleplon • Sleep latency: decrease ($P<.001$) • Total sleep time: increase ($P<.001$) Zolpidem • Sleep latency: decrease ($P<.001$) • Total sleep time: increase ($P<.001$)
Conclusions	• Zaleplon (10 mg and 20 mg), used in the middle of the night 4 h before arising shortens sleep onset • No evidence of impairment of next day performance	• Zaleplon 10 mg and zolpidem 10 mg shorten sleep latency and lengthen sleep duration after dosing, administered during experimental nocturnal awakening • Residual sedation not detected 4 h after zaleplon 10 mg • Residual sedation detected with zolpidem 10 mg $\leq$7 h after treatment • Zaleplon may be an appropriate treatment when patients awaken during the night and have difficulty reinitiating sleep

Abbreviations: CRT, choice reaction time; DSST, Digit Symbol Substitution Test.

Table 6 Zaleplon in primary insomnia	
	Walsh et al,[99] 2000
Study design	Double-blind parallel group placebo-controlled
Number of patients	113
Entry criteria	Primary insomnia
Number of drug evaluation nights	35 nights; baseline, randomization wk 1–5, first 2 nights after treatment discontinuation
Dosage (mg)	Placebo; zaleplon 10
Assessment of sleep	Polysomnography Self-reports
Subjective results	• Sleep latency: decrease (all weeks) ($P \leq .036$) • Tolerance: absent • Rebound insomnia: absent
Objective results	• Sleep latency: decrease (all weeks) ($P \leq .031$) • Total sleep time: inconsistent
Conclusion	• Zaleplon 10 mg effective in treating sleep onset insomnia over a period of 35 nights • Minimal evidence of undesired effects

duration of action and rapid elimination, risks of residual hangover effects are minimized.[103] Zaleplon can be used to combat sleep disturbances at high altitudes.[29] Morera and colleagues[104] have shown zaleplon to increase nocturnal melatonin secretion without increasing daytime levels; this action on melatonin warrants more definitive investigations to determine if zaleplon offers any advantage to circadian rhythm sleep disorders.

Cautions

Cautious use is recommended in major depressive disorder, because it may exacerbate depression.[105] Zaleplon is classified in category C for use in pregnancy. Animal studies showed reduced prenatal and postnatal fetal growth at 49 times the recommended human dose. No controlled human studies have been conducted; therefore, use should be based on possible fetal risk versus maternal benefit. Despite reports of its rapid disappearance from breast milk, use during breastfeeding is best avoided or requires close

monitoring of mother and infant, because there is only limited information on potential risks.[106]

Abuse

Zaleplon carries risks of recreational abuse. It can be insufflated, producing a rapid onset of effects. Being ultra–short acting, it allows for a quicker means of achieving a high. This high lasts for a short period even at the highest doses. Hallucinations and anterograde amnesia are common consequences of abuse, resulting in a loss of ability to monitor increased use and abuse.[107,108] Use should be avoided in patients with a recent history of recreational drug or alcohol abuse and close monitoring if abuse history is remote.

Adverse Effects

Headaches are the most commonly reported side effect, with fewer reports of nausea, myalgia, and abdominal pain. Ability to drive, tested within 4 hours of drug administration, was found unaffected,[109] indicating a lack of residual sedation.[110] It has been reported that individuals receiving zaleplon are less likely to be involved in motor vehicle accidents.[111,112] Memory, learning, and psychomotor function assessed the next day are unaffected at therapeutic doses.[109,113] Fry and colleagues[97] showed that tolerance did not develop with zaleplon over 1 month of treatment. Abrupt withdrawal of drug does not produce a significant withdrawal reaction, allowing as needed use.[114] Research suggests that tolerance and rebound effects with zaleplon are less frequent than with other Z-drugs.[115] Acute intoxication with zaleplon results in drowsiness, blurred speech, ataxia, tachycardia, dizziness, confusion, and vomiting. Treatment is primarily symptomatic.[116,117] There have been case reports of overdose being associated with sleep walking and complex behavior,[118,119] although zaleplon is generally considered to have a lower frequency of sleep-related confusional behaviors than zolpidem or triazolam.

ZOPICLONE AND ESZOPICLONE

Zopiclone is a cyclopyrrolone non-BzRA. Preclinical studies have reported that S-zopiclone, (eg, eszopiclone), is more active than R-zopiclone at the benzodiazepine receptor complex and is responsible for most of the hypnotic effect.[120–122] Eszopiclone has a single chiral center with an S(+) configuration.[123] Both drugs bind significantly to benzodiazepine receptor subtypes sites at α_1, α_2, α_3, and α_5 of the GABA$_A$ complex, enhancing actions of GABA to produce therapeutic and adverse effects.[124] Because zopiclone is not available in the United States, subsequent discussion focuses on eszopiclone. In several studies of normal individuals, Monti and colleagues[125] described the effects of eszopiclone on sleep parameters (shorter sleep onset latency, fewer wakes after sleep onset, greater sleep efficiency, and improved daytime functioning), findings comparable with Rosenberg and colleagues.[126–130]

Pharmacology

As reviewed in **Table 1**, eszopiclone administered orally is rapidly absorbed. Eszopiclone undergoes extensive hepatic metabolism. CYP system inducers and inhibitors affect the biotransformation of eszopiclone; dose adjustments are required during concomitant treatment. Eszopiclone is weakly plasma protein bound, and consequently, its absorption and distribution are minimally affected by other drugs competing for protein binding sites. This factor has resulted in a lowered probability for drug interactions with drugs that strongly bind to plasma proteins.[131] Special recommendations exist for severe hepatic impairment, with doses beginning at 1 mg as systemic exposure in these patients is doubled.[132] On the other hand, no dose adjustments are required for mild to moderate hepatic impairment or mild, moderate, or severe renal insufficiency.[123]

Indications/Uses

Eszopiclone is approved for long-term therapy for sleep initiation and sleep maintenance in patients with transient[130] and chronic primary insomnia.[125,129,133–135] Rosenberg and colleagues[130] assessed the effect of eszopiclone on transient insomnia in healthy adults (**Table 7**). Zammit and colleagues[129] and Roth and colleagues[133] investigated the effects of eszopiclone in chronic primary insomnia (**Table 8**). Recommended dose for adults aged 18 to 64 years is 2 mg for onset insomnia and 3 mg for sleep maintenance problems. Metabolic clearance of eszopiclone is reduced in the elderly ($\geq$65 years), with initial dosing recommended at 2 mg, with further reduction to 1 mg if sleep onset insomnia is the only presenting complaint.[136]

In double-blind, placebo-controlled trials, eszopiclone improved comorbid insomnia in major depression and generalized anxiety without interfering with the therapeutic efficacy of SSRI treatment.[137,138] Perimenopausal and early postmenopausal women with insomnia using eszopiclone showed significant improvements in sleep, mood, menopause-related symptoms, and quality of life.[139] Eszopiclone does not worsen

Table 7 Eszopiclone use in transient insomnia	
	Rosenberg et al,[130] 2005
Study design	Randomized double-blind placebo-controlled multicenter
Number of patients	436 healthy adults
Entry criteria	Transient insomnia (first night effect)
Number of drug evaluation nights	1
Dosage (mg)	Placebo; eszopiclone 1, 3, 3.5
Assessment of sleep	Polysomnography Self-reports
Subjective results	$P\leq$.05 • Sleep latency: decrease (1–3.5 mg) • WASO: decrease (3–3.5 mg) • Total sleep time: increase (2–3.5 mg) • Quality of sleep: increase (2–3.5 mg)
Objective results	$P\leq$.05 • NREM sleep latency: decrease (2–3.5 mg) • WASO: decrease (1–3.5 mg) • Stage 1 sleep: decrease (3.5 mg) • Stage 2 sleep: increase (3.5 mg) • REM sleep: decrease (3.5 mg)
Conclusion	• All doses were more effective than placebo and well tolerated

$P\leq$.05, significantly different from placebo.
Abbreviations: NREM, non–rapid eye movement; REM; rapid eye movement; WASO, wake after sleep onset.
Data from Monti JM, Pandi-Perumal SR. Eszopiclone: its use in the treatment of insomnia. Neuropsychiatr Dis Treat 2007;3(4):441–53.

sleep-disordered breathing and may assist adaptation to the inconvenience of sleep testing and continuous positive airway pressure (CPAP) titration,[140] potentially improving adherence to CPAP therapy.[141] Pollack and colleagues[142] reported a short-term improvement in overall posttraumatic stress disorder severity and associated sleep disturbance, but further investigation was recommended. Improvements in subjective measures of sleep and pain in insomniacs with comorbid rheumatoid arthritis and mucositis secondary to hematologic carcinomas have been described.[143,144]

Table 8
Eszopiclone use in chronic primary insomnia

	Zammit et al,[129] 2004	Roth et al,[133] 2005
Study design	Randomized double-blind placebo-controlled multicenter	Randomized double-blind placebo-controlled for 6 mo then open label for 6 mo
Number of patients	308 (95% completed the study)	360 (111 switched to open label after double-blind placebo)
Entry criteria	DSM-IV criteria for primary insomnia	Sleep duration <6.5 h/night or sleep latency >30 min/night
Number of drug evaluation nights	44 nights	Double-blind placebo (6 mo)　　　Open label (6 mo)
Dosage (mg)	Placebo; eszopiclone 2, 3	Placebo; eszopiclone 3　　　Eszopiclone 3
Assessment of sleep	PSG: nights 1, 15, 29 Self-reports: nights 1, 15, 29, 43/44	Self-reports: monthly (final double-blind month used as baseline for efficacy analyses of open-label period)
Subjective results	$P \leq .05$: • Sleep latency: decrease (2–3 mg) • WASO: decrease (3 mg) • Total sleep time: increase (2–3 mg) • Quality of sleep: increase (2–3 mg) • Rebound insomnia: present on the first night after discontinuing 2 mg of drug • Tolerance: absent	No placebo comparisons: $P \leq .0001$ all monthly end points: • Sleep latency: decrease • WASO: decrease • Number of awakenings: decrease • Total sleep time: increase • Quality of sleep: increase • Daytime functioning: improved • Daytime alertness: improved • Sense of physical well-being: improved • Tolerance: absent
Objective results	$P \leq .05$: • NREM sleep latency: decrease (2–3 mg) • WASO: decrease (3 mg) • Stage 2 sleep: increase (2–3 mg)	
Conclusions	• Better PSG (to night 29) and patient-reported (to night 44) sleep • No tolerance or rebound insomnia • No detrimental effects on next day psychomotor performance	• Significant improvements in sleep and daytime function in those switched from double-blind placebo to open label, which were sustained throughout open label for those receiving previous double-blind eszopiclone • Eszopiclone well tolerated

$P \leq .05/.0001$, significantly different from placebo.
Abbreviations: DSM-IV, Diagnostic and Statistical Manual of Mental Disorders, Fourth Edition; NREM, non-rapid eye movement; PSG, polysomnography; WASO, wake after sleep onset.
Adapted from Monti JM, Pandi-Perumal SR. Eszopiclone: its use in the treatment of insomnia. Neuropsychiatr Dis Treat 2007;3(4):441–53.

Cautions/Abuse

Eszopiclone is assigned to category C for use in pregnancy. Use in nursing mothers should be monitored with great care, because excretion in human milk has not been studied.[145] Scharf[146] reported that eszopiclone at doses of 6 and 12 mg produced euphoria similar to that of 20 mg of diazepam in patients with known dependence on benzodiazepines. In individuals free of polydrug abuse, addictive potential of eszopiclone is unknown but is presumed to be low. Classification of eszopiclone is schedule IV as a controlled substance in the United States.

Adverse Effects

Eszopiclone has fewer anticholinergic side effects than racemic zopiclone and is well tolerated.[120] A common complaint is an unpleasant, metallic taste.[125,147] Other reported effects include dry mouth, gastrointestinal discomfort, headaches, dizziness, and somnolence.[125] Driving skills and cognition assessed on the day after eszopiclone administration were found to be unimpaired.[148] Neuropsychiatric adverse effects mentioned in premarketing data include increased risk for depression, with risks for suicide, agitation, aggression, and transient auditory and visual hallucinations with eszopiclone.[149,150] Memory impairment after long-term use in chronic insomniacs was minimal.[128,129] Decreased sexual desire may be observed.

There is some question about zopiclone and eszopiclone having some potential carcinogenic and mutagenic effects. Stebbing and colleagues[151] presented an uncontrolled case series of the incidence of cancer after eszopiclone prescription, recommending further research. Tolerance or dependence with eszopiclone at 6 months of blinded study and another 6 months of open-label monitoring was not observed.[128,133,136,152] Abrupt discontinuation should be avoided if used for more than 2 weeks to lessen withdrawal symptoms. Overdose has resulted in dulled mental status, ST elevation on electrocardiography, coronary vasospasm, troponemia, ventricular fibrillation, cardiac arrest,[153] and prolonged coma.[154] Treatment should include standard resuscitative and supportive measures.

RATIONALE OF DECREASED DOSE RECOMMENDATIONS FOR ZOLPIDEM OR OTHER SEDATIVE-HYPNOTIC AGENTS IN WOMEN

The recommendations from the FDA for lower dosing in women were made after driving simulation and laboratory studies showed gender differences in performance based on serum plasma levels. Fifteen percent (15%) of 250 women and 3% of 250 men in a study of 250 men and 250 women showed increased levels of zolpidem (>50 ng/mL) 8 hours after dosing. Data have shown that blood levels of greater than 50 ng/mL of zolpidem can impair the ability to drive, thereby increasing the incidence of motor vehicular accidents. Similar trials involving the extended release forms of zolpidem have been described by the FDA, showing 15% of women and 5% of men with 8-hour postdosing zolpidem levels of greater than 50 ng/mL. However, age has an impact, because 10% of both elderly men and women were found to have greater than 50 ng/mL of zolpidem.[155] It is presumed that the gender differences can be explained by the influence of testosterone on metabolism through the cytochrome P450 system.[156] Initial therapeutic dosages should be lower in women, even although women have a higher incidence and prevalence of chronic insomnia.

OTHER BENZODIAZEPINELIKE AGENTS

Indiplon was a pyrazolopyrimidine, nonbenzodiazepine GABA agonist in IR and MR formulations; indication was sought for primary insomnia but it did not receive final FDA approval. It binds selectively to the α_1 subunit compared with α_2, α_3, and α_5 subunits.[157] The CYP3A4/5 enzyme primarily accounts for the formation of 60% to 70% of metabolites.[158,159] Indiplon attains peak plasma levels in 0.73 hours and 0.82 hours and has a half-life of 1.97 hours and 1.71 hours in men and women, respectively.[160] Indiplon follows a dose-dependent linear increase in area under the curve as well as a proportional dose-dependent increase to maximum concentration.[161] The commonly cited adverse drug reactions include headache, gastrointestinal upset, dizziness, and upper respiratory infections.[162–166] The FDA deemed indiplon approvable in 2007 with provisos, but the company discontinued development in the United States.

Gaboxadol or THIP (4, 5, 6, 7-tetrahydroisoxazolo[4,5-c]pyridine-3-ol) is a sedative-hypnotic agent that preferentially binds to the $\alpha_4\delta$ subunit, being unique as a selective extrasynaptic agonist of the δ-containing $GABA_A$ receptor subtype in the thalamus, dentate gyrus, cerebellum, and cortex.[167–171] Animal studies found that the main thalamic pathway known to regulate the sleep-wake cycle and transmitted sensory inputs to the cerebral cortex is believed to be the primary target for gaboxadol. However, within the same circuitry, gaboxadol may in addition interfere with the alternative pathway that bypasses the thalamus to activate both cortical and lateral hypothalamic neurons.[170,172] Gaboxadol acts by binding to the sleep-promoting $\alpha_4\delta$ subunit of $GABA_A$ of the VLPO nucleus.[173] Gaboxadol increased the proportion of non–rapid eye movement sleep, in particular slow wave sleep, without suppressing rapid eye movement sleep.[174–178] Gaboxadol is no longer in clinical development for the treatment of insomnia, based on an assessment of its overall clinical profile in phase 3 trials, including limited or variable efficacy and the occurrence of psychiatric side effects at supratherapeutic doses during an abuse liability study with drug abusers.[179]

SUMMARY

Benzodiazepine receptor agonists such as zolpidem, zaleplon, and eszopiclone show favorable efficacy and safety in double-blind, placebo-controlled trials for transient and chronic insomnia, whether of primary and comorbid origin. Management of chronic insomnia requires assessment for underlying causes through comprehensive assessment of biological, psychological, and lifestyle factors. Practice guidelines recommend cognitive-behavioral therapy as first line, and when deemed appropriate, pharmacologic intervention with a non-BzRA (or ramelteon). Zolpidem (5 and 10 mg), zaleplon (5, 10, and 20 mg) and eszopiclone (2 or 3 mg) at hour of sleep improve sleep onset and efficiency when compared with placebo. Zolpidem CR and eszopiclone taken at lights out maintain sleep through at least 5 to 6 hours of sleep. Zaleplon (5 mg and 10 mg) and sublingual zolpidem IR (1.75 mg for women and 3.5 mg for men) have been approved to be used on awakening if there are 4 or more hours before arising for the day. Because onset of action is similar among the agents, half-life differentiates 1 Z-drug from another. As the shortest acting, zaleplon has the advantage of little hangover and MOTN dosing, although a dose of 10 or 20 mg is often needed in patients with greater hyperarousal. Zolpidem CR or eszopiclone have different binding characteristics of receptor subtypes and likely have some differences that do not make them equivalent hypnotic agents. The receptor subtype binding differences likely explain the higher rate of confusional arousals and sleep-related behavior of zolpidem. Strategies of management of chronic insomnia have included nightly or intermittent (2 or 3 times per week) dosing. Eszopiclone and zolpidem have also been studied to treat comorbid insomnia of major depression or generalized anxiety. For the foreseeable future, the Z-drugs will continue to be the principal pharmaceuticals to improve chronic insomnia.

REFERENCES

1. Schutte-Rodin S, Broch L, Buysse D, et al. Clinical guideline for the evaluation and management of chronic insomnia in adults. J Clin Sleep Med 2008;4(5):487–504.
2. Yules RB, Freedman DX, Chandler KA. The effect of ethyl alcohol on man's electroencephalographic sleep cycle. Electroencephalogr Clin Neurophysiol 1966;20(2):109–11.
3. Sourkes TL. Early clinical neurochemistry of CNS-active drugs. Chloral hydrate. Mol Chem Neuropathol 1992;17(1):21–30.
4. Sourkes TL. Early clinical neurochemistry of CNS-active drugs. Bromides. Mol Chem Neuropathol 1991;14(2):131–42.
5. Nemeroff CB, Putnam JS. Barbiturates and similarly acting substances. In: Sadock B, Sadock V, editors. Kaplan & Sadock's comprehensive textbook of psychiatry. 8th edition. Philadelphia, PA: Lippincott Williams & Wilkins; 2005. p. 2775–81.
6. Harrison NL. Mechanisms of sleep induction by GABA(A) receptor agonists. J Clin Psychiatry 2007;68(Suppl 5):6–12.
7. Arbilla S, Depoortere H, George P, et al. Pharmacological profile of the imidazopyridine zolpidem at benzodiazepine receptors and electrocorticogram in rats. Naunyn Schmiedebergs Arch Pharmacol 1985;330(3):248–51.
8. Perrais D, Ropert N. Effect of zolpidem on miniature IPSCs and occupancy of postsynaptic GABAA receptors in central synapses. J Neurosci 1999; 19(2):578–88.
9. Salvà P, Costa J. Clinical pharmacokinetics and pharmacodynamics of zolpidem. Therapeutic implications. Clin Pharmacokinet 1995;29(3):142–53.
10. Langer SZ, Arbilla S, Scatton B, et al. Receptors involved in the mechanism of action of zolpidem. In: Sauvanet JP, Langer SZ, Morselli PL, editors. Imidazopyridines in sleep disorders. New York: Raven; 1988. p. 55–69.
11. Pritchett DB, Seeburg PH. Gamma-aminobutyric acidA receptor alpha 5-subunit creates novel type II benzodiazepine receptor pharmacology. J Neurochem 1990;54(5):1802–4.
12. Smith AJ, Alder L, Silk J, et al. Effect of alpha subunit on allosteric modulation of ion channel function in stably expressed human recombinant gamma-aminobutyric acid(A) receptors determined using (36)Cl ion flux. Mol Pharmacol 2001;59(5):1108–18.
13. Holm KJ, Goa KL. Zolpidem: an update of its pharmacology, therapeutic efficacy and tolerability in the treatment of insomnia. Drugs 2000; 59(4):865–89.

14. Swainston HT, Keating GM. Zolpidem: a review of its use in the management of insomnia. CNS Drugs 2005;19(1):65–89.

15. Pichard L, Gillet G, Bonfils C, et al. Oxidative metabolism of zolpidem by human liver cytochrome P450S. Drug Metab Dispos 1995;23(11):1253–62.

16. Von Moltke LL, Greenblatt DJ, Granda BW, et al. Zolpidem metabolism in vitro: responsible cytochromes, chemical inhibitors, and in vivo correlations. Br J Clin Pharmacol 1999;48(1):89–97.

17. Merlotti L, Roehrs T, Koshorek G, et al. The dose effects of zolpidem on the sleep of healthy normals. J Clin Psychopharmacol 1989;9(1):9–14.

18. Monti JM. Effect of zolpidem on sleep in insomniac patients. Eur J Clin Pharmacol 1989;36(5):461–6.

19. Scharf MB, Roth T, Vogel GW, et al. A multicenter, placebo-controlled study evaluating zolpidem in the treatment of chronic insomnia. J Clin Psychiatry 1994;55(5):192–9.

20. Monti JM, Monti D, Estévez F, et al. Sleep in patients with chronic primary insomnia during long-term zolpidem administration and after its withdrawal. Int Clin Psychopharmacol 1996;11(4): 255–63.

21. Walsh JK, Roth T, Randazzo A, et al. Eight weeks of non-nightly use of zolpidem for primary insomnia. Sleep 2000;23(8):1087–96.

22. Perlis ML, McCall WV, Krystal AD, et al. Long-term, non-nightly administration of zolpidem in the treatment of patients with primary insomnia. J Clin Psychiatry 2004;65(8):1128–37.

23. Weinling E, McDougall S, Andre F, et al. Pharmacokinetic profile of a new modified release formulation of zolpidem designed to improve sleep maintenance. Fundam Clin Pharmacol 2006; 20(4):397–403.

24. Krystal AD, Erman M, Zammit GK, et al. Long-term efficacy and safety of zolpidem extended-release 12.5 mg, administered 3 to 7 nights per week for 24 weeks, in patients with chronic primary insomnia: a 6-month, randomized, double-blind, placebo-controlled, parallel-group, multicenter study. Sleep 2008;31(1):79–90.

25. Walsh JK, Soubrane C, Roth T. Efficacy and safety of zolpidem extended release in elderly primary insomnia patients. Am J Geriatr Psychiatry 2008; 16(1):44–57.

26. Roth T, Roehrs T, Vogel G. Zolpidem in the treatment of transient insomnia: a double-blind, randomized comparison with placebo. Sleep 1995;18(4):246–51.

27. Asnis GM, Chakraburtty A, DuBoff EA, et al. Zolpidem for persistent insomnia in SSRI-treated depressed patients. J Clin Psychiatry 1999; 60(10):668–76.

28. Available at: http://www.e-publishing.af.mil/shared/media/epubs/AFSOCI48-101.pdf. Accessed December 10, 2012.

29. Beaumont M, Batéjat D, Piérard C, et al. Zaleplon and zolpidem objectively alleviate sleep disturbances in mountaineers at a 3,613 meter altitude. Sleep 2007;30(11):1527–33.

30. Hajak G, Geisler P. Experience with zolpidem 'as needed' in primary care settings. CNS Drugs 2004;18(Suppl 1):35–40.

31. Lévy P, Massuel M, Gérard DA. 'As-needed' prescription of zolpidem for insomnia in routine general practice. Clin Drug Investig 2004;24(11):625–32.

32. Roth T, Hull SG, Lankford DA, et al. Low-dose sublingual zolpidem tartrate is associated with dose-related improvement in sleep onset and duration in insomnia characterized by middle-of-the-night (MOTN) awakenings. Sleep 2008;31(9):1277–84.

33. Depoortere H, Zivkovic B, Lloyd KG, et al. Zolpidem, a novel nonbenzodiazepine hypnotic. I. Neuropharmacological and behavioral effects. J Pharmacol Exp Ther 1986;237(2):649–58.

34. Ambien (zolpidem tartrate) tablet prescribing information. Bridgewater (NJ): Sanofi-Aventis; 2007.

35. Ambien CR (zolpidem tartrate) extended-release tablet prescribing information. Bridgewater (NJ): Sanofi-Aventis; 2007.

36. Wikner BN, Källén B. Are hypnotic benzodiazepine receptor agonists teratogenic in humans? J Clin Psychopharmacol 2011;31(3):356–9.

37. Wang LH, Lin HC, Lin CC, et al. Increased risk of adverse pregnancy outcomes in women receiving zolpidem during pregnancy. Clin Pharmacol Ther 2010;88(3):369–74.

38. Sharma A, Sayeed N, Khees CR, et al. High dose zolpidem induced fetal neural tube defects. Curr Drug Saf 2011;6(2):128–9.

39. Pons G, Francoual C, Guillet P, et al. Zolpidem excretion in breast milk. Eur J Clin Pharmacol 1989;37(3):245–8.

40. Liappas IA, Malitas PN, Dimopoulos NP, et al. Zolpidem dependence case series: possible neurobiological mechanisms and case management. J Psychopharmacol 2003;17(1):131–5.

41. Gericke CA, Ludolph AC. Chronic abuse of zolpidem. JAMA 1994;272(22):1721–2.

42. Cohen L, Chaaban B, Habert MO. Transient improvement of aphasia with zolpidem. N Engl J Med 2004;350(9):949–50.

43. Clauss R, Nel W. Drug induced arousal from the permanent vegetative state. NeuroRehabilitation 2006;21(1):23–8.

44. Whyte J, Myers R. Incidence of clinically significant responses to zolpidem among patients with disorders of consciousness: a preliminary placebo controlled trial. American Journal Physical Medicine Rehabilitation 2009;88(5):410–8.

45. Hall SD, Yamawaki N, Fisher AE, et al. GABA(A) alpha-1 subunit mediated desynchronization of elevated low frequency oscillations alleviates

specific dysfunction in stroke–a case report. Clinical Neurophysiology 2010;121(4):549–55.

46. Nyakale NE, Clauss RP, Nel W, et al. Clinical and brain SPECT scan response to zolpidem in patients after brain damage. Arzneimittelforschung 2010; 60(4):177–81.

47. Machado C, Estévez M, Pérez-Nellar J, et al. Autonomic, EEG, and behavioral arousal signs in a PVS case after zolpidem intake. Canadian Journal Neurological Sciences 2011;38(2):341–4.

48. Clauss RP, Güldenpfennig WM, Nel HW, et al. Extraordinary arousal from semi-comatose state on zolpidem. A case report. S Afr Med J 2000; 90(1):68–72.

49. Brefel-Courbon C, Payoux P, Ory F, et al. Clinical and imaging evidence of zolpidem effect in hypoxic encephalopathy. Ann Neurol 2007;62(1):102–5.

50. Cohen SI, Duong TT. Increased arousal in a patient with anoxic brain injury after administration of zolpidem. Am J Phys Med Rehabil 2008;87(3):229–31.

51. Shames JL, Ring H. Transient reversal of anoxic brain injury-related minimally conscious state after zolpidem administration: a case report. Arch Phys Med Rehabil 2008;89(2):386–8.

52. Snyman N, Egan JR, London K, et al. Zolpidem for persistent vegetative state–a placebo-controlled trial in pediatrics. Neuropediatrics 2010;41(5): 223–7.

53. Garretto NS, Bueri JA, Rey RD, et al. Improvement of blepharospasm with zolpidem. Mov Disord 2004;19(8):967–8.

54. Wang WT, Chen YY, Wu SL, et al. Zolpidem dramatically improved motor and speech function in a patient with central pontine myelinolysis. Eur J Neurol 2007;14(10):e9–10.

55. Thomas P, Rascle C, Mastain B, et al. Test for catatonia with zolpidem. Lancet 1997;349(9053):702.

56. Clauss R, Sathekge M, Nel W. Transient improvement of spinocerebellar ataxia with zolpidem. N Engl J Med 2004;351(5):511–2.

57. Shadan FF, Poceta JS, Kline LE. Zolpidem for post-anoxic spasticity. South Med J 2004;97(8):791–2.

58. Bezerra ML, Martínez JV. Zolpidem in restless legs syndrome. Eur Neurol 2002;48(3):180–1.

59. Daniele A, Moro E, Bentivoglio AR. Zolpidem in progressive supranuclear palsy. N Engl J Med 1999;341(7):543–4.

60. Daniele A, Albanese A, Gainotti G, et al. Zolpidem in Parkinson's disease. Lancet 1997;349(9060): 1222–3.

61. Růžicka E, Roth J, Jech R, et al. Subhypnotic doses of zolpidem oppose dopaminergic-induced dyskinesia in Parkinson's disease. Mov Disord 2000;15(4):734–5.

62. Farver DK, Khan MH. Zolpidem for antipsychotic-induced parkinsonism. Ann Pharmacother 2001; 35(4):435–7.

63. Evidente VG. Zolpidem improves dystonia in "Lubag" or X-linked dystonia-parkinsonism syndrome. Neurology 2002;58(4):662–3.

64. Shyu C, Burke K, Souweidane MM, et al. Novel use of zolpidem in cerebellar mutism syndrome. J Pediatr Hematol Oncol 2011;33(2):148–9.

65. Tsai MJ, Tsai YH, Huang YB. Compulsive activity and anterograde amnesia after zolpidem use. Clin Toxicol (Phila) 2007;45(2):179–81.

66. Tsai JH, Yang P, Chen CC, et al. Zolpidem-induced amnesia and somnambulism: rare occurrences? Eur Neuropsychopharmacol 2009;19(1):74–6.

67. Praplan-Pahud J, Forster A, Gamulin Z, et al. Preoperative sedation before regional anaesthesia: comparison between zolpidem, midazolam and placebo. Br J Anaesth 1990;64(6):670–4.

68. Inagaki T, Miyaoka T, Tsuji S, et al. Adverse reactions to zolpidem: case reports and a review of the literature. Prim Care Companion J Clin Psychiatry 2010;12(6). pii:PCC.09r00849.

69. Canaday BR. Amnesia possibly associated with zolpidem administration. Pharmacotherapy 1996; 16(4):687–9.

70. Drover D, Lemmens H, Naidu S, et al. Pharmacokinetics, pharmacodynamics, and relative pharmacokinetic/pharmacodynamic profiles of zaleplon and zolpidem. Clin Ther 2000;22(12):1443–61.

71. Toner LC, Tsambiras BM, Catalano G, et al. Central nervous system side effects associated with zolpidem treatment. Clin Neuropharmacol 2000; 23(1):54–8.

72. Howell MJ, Schenck CH, Crow SJ. A review of nighttime eating disorders. Sleep Med Rev 2009; 13(1):23–34.

73. Harazin J, Berigan TR. Zolpidem tartrate and somnambulism. Mil Med 1999;164(9):669–70.

74. Mendelson WB. Sleepwalking associated with zolpidem. J Clin Psychopharmacol 1994;14(2):150.

75. Sharma A, Dewan VK. A case report of zolpidem-induced somnambulism. Prim Care Companion J Clin Psychiatry 2005;7(2):74.

76. Sansone RA, Sansone LA. Zolpidem, somnambulism, and nocturnal eating. Gen Hosp Psychiatry 2008;30(1):90–1.

77. Yang W, Dollear M, Muthukrishnan SR. One rare side effect of zolpidem–sleepwalking: a case report. Arch Phys Med Rehabil 2005;86(6):1265–6.

78. Max HP, Kushan R, Brian MW, et al. Effects of eszopiclone and zolpidem on sleep-wake behavior, anxiety-like behavior and contextual memory in rats. Behav Brain Res 2010;210(1):54–66.

79. Vermeeren A. Residual effects of hypnotics: epidemiology and clinical implications. CNS Drugs 2004; 18(5):297–328.

80. Bocca ML, Marie S, Lelong-Boulouard V, et al. Zolpidem and zopiclone impair similarly monotonous driving performance after a single nighttime

intake in aged subjects. Psychopharmacology (Berl) 2011;214(3):699–706.

81. Olubodun JO, Ochs HR, von Moltke LL, et al. Pharmacokinetic properties of zolpidem in elderly and young adults: possible modulation by testosterone in men. Br J Clin Pharmacol 2003;56(3):297–304.

82. Wang PS, Bohn RL, Glynn RJ, et al. Zolpidem use and hip fractures in older people. J Am Geriatr Soc 2001;49(12):1685–90.

83. Staner L, Ertlé S, Boeijinga P, et al. Next-day residual effects of hypnotics in DSM-IV primary insomnia: a driving simulator study with simultaneous electroencephalogram monitoring. Psychopharmacology (Berl) 2005;181(4):790–8.

84. Mattoo SK, Gaur N, Das PP. Zolpidem withdrawal delirium. Indian J Pharmacol 2011;43(6):729–30.

85. Zosel A, Osterberg EC, Mycyk MB. Zolpidem misuse with other medications or alcohol frequently results in intensive care unit admission. Am J Ther 2011;18(4):305–8.

86. Quaglio G, Lugoboni F, Fornasiero A, et al. Dependence on zolpidem: two case reports of detoxification with flumazenil infusion. Int Clin Psychopharmacol 2005;20(5):285–7.

87. Rappa LR, Larose-Pierre M, Payne DR, et al. Detoxification from high dose zolpidem using diazepam. Ann Pharmacother 2004;38(4):590–4.

88. Kuzniar TJ, Balagani R, Radigan KA, et al. Coma with absent brainstem reflexes resulting from zolpidem overdose. Am J Ther 2010;17(5):e172–4.

89. Hamad A, Sharma N. Acute zolpidem overdose leading to coma and respiratory failure. Intensive Care Med 2001;27(7):1239.

90. Lheureux P, Debailleul G, De Witte O, et al. Zolpidem intoxication mimicking narcotic overdose: response to flumazenil. Hum Exp Toxicol 1990; 9(2):105–7.

91. Oulis P, Nakkas G, Masdrakis VG. Pregabalin in zolpidem dependence and withdrawal. Clin Neuropharmacol 2011;34(2):90–1.

92. Elie R, Rüther E, Farr I, et al. Sleep latency is shortened during 4 weeks of treatment with zaleplon, a novel nonbenzodiazepine hypnotic. J Clin Psychiatry 1999;60(8):536–44.

93. Lake BG, Ball SE, Kao J, et al. Metabolism of zaleplon by human liver: evidence for involvement of aldehyde oxidase. Xenobiotica 2002; 32(10):835–47.

94. Renwick AB, Mistry H, Ball SE, et al. Metabolism of zaleplon by human hepatic microsomal cytochrome P450 isoforms. Xenobiotica 1998;28(4): 337–48.

95. Hedner J, Yaeche R, Emilien G, et al. Zaleplon shortens subjective sleep latency and improves subjective sleep quality in elderly patients with insomnia. Int J Geriatr Psychiatry 2000;15(8): 704–12.

96. Richardson GS, Roth T, Kramer JA. Management of insomnia–the role of zaleplon. MedGenMed 2002; 4(1):9.

97. Fry J, Scharf M, Mangano R, et al. Zaleplon improves sleep without producing rebound effects in outpatients with insomnia. Int Clin Psychopharmacol 2000;15(3):141–52.

98. Stone BM, Turner C, Mills SL, et al. Noise-induced sleep maintenance insomnia: hypnotic and residual effects of zaleplon. Br J Clin Pharmacol 2002; 53(2):196–202.

99. Walsh JK, Vogel GW, Scharf M, et al. A five week, polysomnographic assessment of zaleplon 10 mg for the treatment of primary insomnia. Sleep Med 2000;1(1):41–9.

100. Zammit GK, Corser B, Doghramji K, et al. Sleep and residual sedation after administration of zaleplon, zolpidem, and placebo during experimental middle-of-the-night-awakening. J Clin Sleep Med 2006;2(4):417–23.

101. Greenblatt DJ, Harmatz JS, Walsh JK, et al. Pharmacokinetic profile of SKP-1041, a modified release formulation of zaleplon. Biopharm Drug Dispos 2011;32(9):489–97.

102. Weitzel KW, Wickman JM, Augustin SG, et al. Zaleplon: a pyrazolopyrimidine sedative-hypnotic agent for the treatment of insomnia. Clin Ther 2000;22(11):1254–67.

103. Wagner J, Wagner ML, Hening WA. Beyond benzodiazepines: alternative pharmacologic agents for the treatment of insomnia. Ann Pharmacother 1998;32(6):680–91.

104. Morera AL, Abreu-Gonzalez P, Henry M. Zaleplon increases nocturnal melatonin secretion in humans. Prog Neuropsychopharmacol Biol Psychiatry 2009; 33(6):1013–6.

105. Kripke DF. Greater incidence of depression with hypnotic use than with placebo. BMC Psychiatry 2007;7:42.

106. Darwish M, Martin PT, Cevallos WH, et al. Rapid disappearance of zaleplon from breast milk after oral administration to lactating women. J Clin Pharmacol 1999;39(7):670–4.

107. Rush CR, Frey JM, Griffiths RR. Zaleplon and triazolam in humans: acute behavioral effects and abuse potential. Psychopharmacology (Berl) 1999;145(1):39–51.

108. Ator NA. Zaleplon and triazolam: drug discrimination, plasma levels, and self-administration in baboons. Drug Alcohol Depend 2000;61(1):55–68.

109. Verster JC, Volkerts ER, Schreuder AH, et al. Residual effects of middle-of-the-night administration of zaleplon and zolpidem on driving ability, memory functions, and psychomotor performance. J Clin Psychopharmacol 2002;22(6):576–83.

110. Walsh JK, Pollak CP, Scharf MB, et al. Lack of residual sedation following middle-of-the-night

zaleplon administration in sleep maintenance insomnia. Clin Neuropharmacol 2000;23(1):17–21.

111. Menzin J, Lang KM, Levy P, et al. A general model of the effects of sleep medications on the risk and cost of motor vehicle accidents and its application to France. Pharmacoeconomics 2001;19(1):69–78.

112. Vermeeren A, Riedel WJ, van Boxtel MP, et al. Differential residual effects of zaleplon and zopiclone on actual driving: a comparison with a low dose of alcohol. Sleep 2002;25(2):224–31.

113. Troy SM, Lucki I, Unruh MA, et al. Comparison of the effects of zaleplon, zolpidem, and triazolam on memory, learning, and psychomotor performance. J Clin Psychopharmacol 2000;20(3):328–37.

114. Israel AG, Kramer JA. Safety of zaleplon in the treatment of insomnia. Ann Pharmacother 2002; 36(5):852–9.

115. Lader MH. Implications of hypnotic flexibility on patterns of clinical use. Int J Clin Pract Suppl 2001;116:14–9.

116. Sein AJ, Chodorowski Z, Hajduk A. Acute intoxication with zaleplon–a case report. Przegl Lek 2007; 64(4–5):310–1.

117. Louis CJ, Fernandez B, Beaumont C, et al. A case of zaleplon overdose. Clin Toxicol (Phila) 2008; 46(8):782.

118. Liskow B, Pikalov A. Zaleplon overdose associated with sleepwalking and complex behavior. J Am Acad Child Adolesc Psychiatry 2004;43(8):927–8.

119. Lange CL. Medication-associated somnambulism. J Am Acad Child Adolesc Psychiatry 2005;44(3): 211–2.

120. Georgiev V. (S)-Zopiclone Sepracor. Curr Opin Investig Drugs 2001;2:271–3.

121. McMahon LR, Jerussi TP, France CP. Stereoselective discriminative stimulus effects of zopiclone in rhesus monkeys. Psychopharmacology 2003;165: 222–8.

122. Carlson JN, Haskew R, Wacker J, et al. Sedative and anxiolytic effects of zopiclone's enantiomers and metabolite. Eur J Pharmacol 2001;415(2–3): 181–9.

123. Najib J. Eszopiclone, a nonbenzodiazepine sedative-hypnotic agent for the treatment of transient and chronic insomnia. Clin Ther 2006;28(4): 491–516.

124. Drover DR. Comparative pharmacokinetics and pharmacodynamics of short-acting hypnosedatives: zaleplon, zolpidem and zopiclone. Clin Pharmacokinet 2004;43(4):227–38.

125. Monti JM, Pandi-Perumal SR. Eszopiclone: its use in the treatment of insomnia. Neuropsychiatr Dis Treat 2007;3(4):441–53.

126. Scharf M, Erman M, Rosenberg R, et al. A 2-week efficacy and safety study of eszopiclone in elderly patients with primary insomnia. Sleep 2005;28(6): 720–7.

127. McCall WV, Erman M, Krystal AD, et al. A polysomnography study of eszopiclone in elderly patients with insomnia. Curr Med Res Opin 2006; 22(9):1633–42.

128. Krystal AD, Walsh JK, Laska E, et al. Sustained efficacy of eszopiclone over 6 months of nightly treatment: results of a randomized, double-blind, placebo-controlled study in adults with chronic insomnia. Sleep 2003;26(7):793–9.

129. Zammit GK, McNabb LJ, Caron J, et al. Efficacy and safety of eszopiclone across 6 weeks of treatment for primary insomnia. Curr Med Res Opin 2004;20(12):1979–91.

130. Rosenberg R, Caron J, Roth T, et al. An assessment of the efficacy and safety of eszopiclone in the treatment of transient insomnia in healthy adults. Sleep Med 2005;6(1):15–22.

131. Laustsen G. Eszopiclone (Lunesta) for treatment of insomnia. Nurse Pract 2005;30(9):67–8.

132. McCrae CS, Ross A, Stripling A, et al. Eszopiclone for late-life insomnia. Clin Interv Aging 2007;2(3): 313–26.

133. Roth T, Walsh JK, Krystal A, et al. An evaluation of the efficacy and safety of eszopiclone over 12 months in patients with chronic primary insomnia. Sleep Med 2005;6(6):487–95.

134. Melton ST, Wood JM, Kirkwood CK. Eszopiclone for insomnia. Ann Pharmacother 2005;39(10):1659–66.

135. Eszopiclone: esopiclone, estorra, S-zopiclone, zopiclone–Sepracor. Drugs R D 2005;6(2):111–5.

136. Lunesta approved labeling text. Marlborough (MA): Sepracor; 2005.

137. Krystal A, Fava M, Rubens R, et al. Evaluation of eszopiclone discontinuation after cotherapy with fluoxetine for insomnia with coexisting depression. J Clin Sleep Med 2007;3(1):48–55.

138. Fava M, McCall WV, Krystal A, et al. Eszopiclone co-administered with fluoxetine in patients with insomnia coexisting with major depressive disorder. Biol Psychiatry 2006;59(11):1052–60.

139. Soares CN, Joffe H, Rubens R, et al. Eszopiclone in patients with insomnia during perimenopause and early postmenopause: a randomized controlled trial. Obstet Gynecol 2006;108(6):1402–10.

140. Lettieri CJ, Quast TN, Eliasson AH, et al. Eszopiclone improves overnight polysomnography and continuous positive airway pressure titration: a prospective, randomized, placebo-controlled trial. Sleep 2008;31(9):1310–6.

141. Lettieri CJ, Collen JF, Eliasson AH, et al. Sedative use during continuous positive airway pressure titration improves subsequent compliance: a randomized, double-blind, placebo-controlled trial. Chest 2009;136(5):1263–8.

142. Pollack MH, Hoge EA, Worthington JJ, et al. Eszopiclone for the treatment of posttraumatic stress disorder and associated insomnia: a

143. Roth T, Price JM, Amato DA, et al. The effect of eszopiclone in patients with insomnia and coexisting rheumatoid arthritis: a pilot study. Prim Care Companion J Clin Psychiatry 2009;11(6):292–301.

144. Dimsdale JE, Ball ED, Carrier E, et al. Effect of eszopiclone on sleep, fatigue, and pain in patients with mucositis associated with hematologic malignancies. Support Care Cancer 2011;19(12):2015–20.

145. Lunesta prescribing information. Marlborough (MA): Sepracor; 2005.

146. Scharf M. Eszopiclone for the treatment of insomnia. Expert Opin Pharmacother 2006;7(3): 345–56.

147. Wadworth AN, McTavish D. Zopiclone. A review of its pharmacological properties and therapeutic efficacy as an hypnotic. Drugs Aging 1993;3(5):441–59.

148. Boyle J, Trick L, Johnsen S, et al. Next-day cognition, psychomotor function, and driving-related skills following nighttime administration of eszopiclone. Hum Psychopharmacol 2008;23(5):385–97.

149. Lunesta (eszopiclone) prescribing information. Marlborough (MA): Sepracor; 2005.

150. Duggal HS. New-onset transient hallucinations possibly due to eszopiclone: a case study. Prim Care Companion J Clin Psychiatry 2007;9(6):468–9.

151. Stebbing J, Waters L, Davies L, et al. Incidence of cancer in individuals receiving chronic zopiclone or eszopiclone requires prospective study. J Clin Oncol 2005;23(31):8134–6.

152. Brielmaier BD. Eszopiclone (Lunesta): a new nonbenzodiazepine hypnotic agent. Proc (Bayl Univ Med Cent) 2006;19(1):54–9.

153. Miller AH, Bruggman AR, Miller MM. Lunesta overdose: ST-elevation coronary vasospasm, troponemia, and ventricular fibrillation arrest. Am J Emerg Med 2006;24(6):741–6.

154. Lovett B, Watts D, Grossman M. Prolonged coma after eszopiclone overdose. Am J Emerg Med 2007;25(6):735.

155. Verster JC, Roth T. Gender differences in highway driving performance after administration of sleep medication: a review of the literature. Traffic Inj Prev 2012;13(3):286–92.

156. Greenblatt DJ, Harmatz JS, von Moltke LL, et al. Comparative kinetics and response to the benzodiazepine agonists triazolam and zolpidem: evaluation of sex-dependent differences. J Pharmacol Exp Ther 2000;293:435–43.

157. Petroski RE, Pomeroy JE, Das R, et al. Indiplon, is a high-affinity positive allosteric modulator with selectivity for α1 subunit-containing GABAA receptors. J Pharmacol Exp Ther 2006;317(1): 369–77.

158. Madan A, Fisher A, Jin L, Chapman D, Bozigian HP. In vitro metabolism of indiplon and an assessment of its drug interaction potential. Xenobiotica 2007;37(7):736–52.

159. Lemon MD, Strain JD, Hegg AM, et al. Indiplon in the management of insomnia. Drug Des Devel Ther 2009;3:131–42.

160. Rogowski R, Garber M, Bozigian H, et al. NBI-34060 (a non-benzodiazepine sedative-hypnotic): lack of a pharmacokinetic gender effect. Sleep 2002;25(Suppl):A415.

161. Bozigian H, Chen TK, Gately N, et al. Indiplon dose-proportional pharmacokinetics. J Clin Pharmacol 2005;45:1078.

162. Scharf MB, Black J, Hull S, et al. Long-term nightly treatment with indiplon in adults with primary insomnia: results of a double-blind, placebo-controlled, 3-month study. Sleep 2007; 30(6):743–52.

163. Walsh JK, Moscovitch A, Burke J, et al. Efficacy and tolerability of indiplon in older adults with primary insomnia. Sleep Med 2007;8(7–8):753–9.

164. Roth T, Zammit GK, Scharf MB, et al. Efficacy and safety of as-needed, post bedtime dosing with indiplon in insomnia patients with chronic difficulty maintaining sleep. Sleep 2007;30(12):1731–8.

165. Rosenberg R, Roth T, Scharf MB, et al. Efficacy and tolerability of indiplon in transient insomnia. J Clin Sleep Med 2007;3(4):374–9.

166. Black J, Burke J, Bell J, et al. Safety and tolerability of long-term treatment with indiplon: results of a randomized 12-month study. Sleep 2006; 29(Suppl):A255.

167. Meera P, Wallner M, Otis TS. Molecular basis for the high THIP/gaboxadol sensitivity of extrasynaptic GABAA receptors. J Neurophysiol 2011;106(4): 2057–64.

168. Ebert B, Wafford KA, Deacon S. Treating insomnia: current and investigational pharmacological approaches. Pharmacol Ther 2006;112(3):612–29.

169. Wafford KA, Ebert B. Gaboxadol–a new awakening in sleep. Curr Opin Pharmacol 2006;6(1):30–6.

170. Belelli D, Peden DR, Rosahl TW, et al. Extrasynaptic GABAA receptors of thalamocortical neurons: a molecular target for hypnotics. J Neurosci 2005; 25(50):11513–20.

171. Orser BA. Extrasynaptic GABAA receptors are critical targets for sedative-hypnotic drugs. J Clin Sleep Med 2006;2(2):S12–8.

172. Saper CB, Chou TC, Scammell TE. The sleep switch: hypothalamic control of sleep and wakefulness. Trends Neurosci 2001;24(12):726–31.

173. Lu J, Greco MA. Sleep circuitry and the hypnotic mechanism of GABAA drugs. J Clin Sleep Med 2006;2(2):S19–26.

174. Deacon S, Staner L, Staner C, et al. Effect of short-term treatment with gaboxadol on sleep maintenance and initiation in patients with primary insomnia. Sleep 2007;30(3):281–7.

175. Lundahl J, Staner L, Staner C, et al. Short-term treatment with gaboxadol improves sleep maintenance and enhances slow wave sleep in adult patients with primary insomnia. Psychopharmacology (Berl) 2007;195:139–46.

176. Walsh JK, Deacon S, Dijk DJ, et al. The selective extrasynaptic GABAA agonist, gaboxadol, improves traditional hypnotic efficacy measures and enhances slow wave activity in a model of transient insomnia. Sleep 2007;30:593–602.

177. Mathias S, Steiger A, Lancel M. The GABA(A) agonist gaboxadol improves the quality of post-nap sleep. Psychopharmacology (Berl) 2001;157: 299–304.

178. Mathias S, Zihl J, Steiger A, et al. Effect of repeated gaboxadol administration on night sleep and next-day performance in healthy elderly subjects. Neuropsychopharmacology 2005;30:833–41.

179. Lundbeck. Discontinuation of development program for gaboxadol in insomnia. Available at: http://www.lundbeck.com/investor/Presentations/Teleconference/Teleconference_gaboxadol_20070328.pdf.3-27-2007. Accessed May 21, 2008.

180. Fernandez C, Maradeix V, Gimenez F, et al. Pharmacokinetics of zopiclone and its enantiomers in Caucasian young healthy volunteers. Drug Metab Dispos 1993;21(6):1125–8.

181. Fernandez C, Martin C, Gimenez F, et al. Clinical pharmacokinetics of zopiclone. Clin Pharmacokinet 1995;29(6):431–41.

182. Noble S, Langtry HD, Lamb HM. Zopiclone. An update of its pharmacology, clinical efficacy and tolerability in the treatment of insomnia. Drugs 1998;55(2):277–302.

183. de Haas SL, Schoemaker RC, van Gerven JM, et al. Pharmacokinetics, pharmacodynamics and the pharmacokinetic/pharmacodynamic relationship of zolpidem in healthy subjects. J Psychopharmacol 2010;24(11):1619–29.

184. Greenblatt DJ, Harmatz JS, Shader RI. Clinical pharmacokinetics of anxiolytics and hypnotics in the elderly: therapeutic considerations. Clin Pharmacokinet 1991;21:165–77, 262–73.

185. von Moltke LL, Abernethy DR, Greenblatt DJ. Kinetics and dynamics of psychotropic drugs in the elderly. In: Salzman C, editor. Clinical geriatric psychopharmacology. Baltimore (MD): Williams & Wilkins; 1998. p. 70–93.

186. Rosen AS, Fournié P, Darwish M, et al. Zaleplon pharmacokinetics and absolute bioavailability. Biopharm Drug Dispos 1999;20(3):171–5.

187. Greenblatt DJ, Harmatz JS, von Moltke LL, et al. Comparative kinetics and dynamics of zaleplon, zolpidem, and placebo. Clin Pharmacol Ther 1998;64(5):553–61.

188. Sanger DJ. The pharmacology and mechanisms of action of new generation, non-benzodiazepine hypnotic agents. CNS Drugs 2004;18(Suppl 1): 9–15.

189. Patat A, Trocherie S, Thebault JJ, et al. EEG profile of intravenous zolpidem in healthy volunteers. Psychopharmacology (Berl) 1994;114(1):138–46.

190. Fernandez C, Maradeix V, Gimenez F, et al. Pharmacokinetics of zopiclone and its enantiomers in Caucasian young healthy volunteers. Drug Metab Dispos 1999;21(6):1125–8.

191. Becquemont L, Mouajjah S, Escaffre O, et al. Cytochrome P-450 3A4 and 2C8 are involved in zopiclone metabolism. Drug Metab Dispos 1999; 27(9):1068–73.

192. Greenblatt DJ, von Moltke LL, Harmatz JS, et al. Kinetic and dynamic interaction study of zolpidem with ketoconazole, itraconazole, and fluconazole. Clin Pharmacol Ther 1998;64(6):661–71.

193. Wang JS, DeVane CL. Pharmacokinetics and drug interactions of the sedative hypnotics. Psychopharmacol Bull 2003;37(1):10–29.

194. Hetta J, Broman JE, Darwish M, et al. Psychomotor effects of zaleplon and thioridazine coadministration. Eur J Clin Pharmacol 2000;56(3):211–7.

195. Koshorek G, Roehrs T, Sicklesteel J, et al. Dose effects of zolpidem on transient insomnia. Sleep Res 1988;17:47.

196. Monti JM, Boussard M, Olivera S, et al. The effect of midazolam on transient insomnia. Eur J Clin Pharmacol 1993;44(6):525–7.

Application of Cognitive Behavioral Therapies for Comorbid Insomnia and Depression

Patricia Haynes, PhD

KEYWORDS

- Insomnia • Depression • Cognitive behavioral therapy

KEY POINTS

- Insomnia and depression are highly comorbid clinical states.
- Key elements of CBT-I include stimulus control therapy, sleep restriction therapy, and cognitive restructuring. CBT-I is highly effective for insomnia and also reduces depression symptoms and depression relapse. Depressed individuals may be more likely to terminate from CBT-I prematurely and may also have some difficulties remaining adherent to the therapy. Those individuals who do complete treatment seem to have a treatment response comparable to nondepressed individuals.
- Key elements of CBT-D include behavioral activation and cognitive restructuring. CBT-D is highly effective for depression and also reduces insomnia symptoms. One study found that residual insomnia after CBT-D does not predict relapse/recurrence above and beyond the impact of residual anxiety symptoms. Studies are necessary to examine whether insomnia moderates CBT-D treatment adherence or response.
- It is recommended that CBT-I therapists incorporate elements of CBT-D into the therapy with depressed patients to address adherence problems caused by motivational deficits, avoidance, and depressogenic automatic thoughts. Cognitive behavioral social rhythm therapy has incorporated principles of both CBT-I and CBT-D.

INTRODUCTION

Insomnia co-occurs frequently with depression. Approximately 80% of depressed individuals experience some form of insomnia symptom.[1] Up to 12% of patients with depression may have insomnia symptoms sufficiently severe enough to warrant a comorbid diagnosis, although it is a predominant characteristic of the symptomology in only 6% of depressed patients.[1] Given the high prevalence with which insomnia co-occurs with depression, insomnia has historically been assumed to be a by-product of depression and hence its inclusion as a symptom of a Major Depressive Episode in the *Diagnostic and Statistical Manual of Mental Disorders, fifth edition*.[2] Studies that have examined the timeframe of the development of the two states have indicated that depression may actually be causally related to insomnia. Insomnia often occurs before depression[3–5] and predicts depression recurrence.[6] Practice parameters put forth by the American Academy of Sleep Medicine now encourage providers to conceptualize insomnia as a comorbid disorder (vs secondary disorder) when associated with depression.[7]

Department of Psychiatry, University of Arizona, 1501 North Campbell Avenue, PO Box 245002, Tucson, AZ 85724-5002, USA
E-mail address: thaynes@email.arizona.edu

Sleep Med Clin 10 (2015) 77–84
http://dx.doi.org/10.1016/j.jsmc.2014.11.006
1556-407X/15/$ – see front matter © 2015 Elsevier Inc. All rights reserved.

This comorbid conceptualization is consistent with temporal data showing that insomnia comorbid with depression is an important intermediate phenotype between pure insomnia and depression.[8] Patients with both insomnia and depression experience a more severe clinical state. As compared with insomnia patients only, insomnia patients with comorbid depression have greater presleep mental arousal, more maladaptive beliefs and attitudes about sleep, more sleep effort, and worse sleep hygiene than insomnia patients without depression.[9,10] Persistent insomnia with depression is associated with suicide[11,12] and an increased tendency to use global attributions for negative events (eg, "This issues creates problems in *all* areas of my life"),[13] a hallmark characteristic of learned helplessness. Disrupted sleep profiles in depression are associated with longer depressive episode duration, a more severe history of depressive illness, a greater number of depressive episodes, and being earlier in the course of a depressive episode.[14]

Altogether, these data are important because they illustrate the necessity of treatment procedures that take both insomnia and depression into account. Cognitive behavioral therapy (CBT) is a well-tested, evidence-based behavioral intervention for depression and insomnia that seems to be at least equal to the effect of medication for each disorder. Relatively few studies have examined the impact of CBT on both disorders. Examination of depression and insomnia outcomes in CBT is important, because it provides a means by which to determine unique ways each version of CBT (CBT for insomnia [CBT-I] and CBT for depression [CBT-D]) address symptoms of the alternate disorder. These data also inform ways that CBTs might need modification to address the comorbid condition.

This article introduces ways that CBTs have been used in depression and insomnia with a focus on the impact each therapy has had on the alternate diagnosis.

COGNITIVE BEHAVIORAL THERAPY FOR INSOMNIA AND DEPRESSION

CBT-I is a well-tested, highly effective evidence-based psychotherapy for insomnia. The three key active components of CBT-I are (1) stimulus control, (2) sleep restriction, and (3) cognitive restructuring, although CBT-I also includes education about sleep, relaxation training, and sleep hygiene (eg, instructions to discontinue caffeine, alcohol, and so forth). The first active component of CBT-I is stimulus control, a behavioral intervention designed to counter the learned association between bed/bedroom and wakefulness.[15] With stimulus control, patients are instructed to retire to bed only when sleepy, use the bed only for sleep and sex, arise from bed if unable to sleep (repetitively throughout the night if necessary), and arise at a regular time each morning. The second active component of CBT-I is sleep restriction, a behavioral intervention that uses the homeostatic sleep drive to consolidate sleep.[16] In sleep restriction therapy, individuals are instructed to reduce their overall time in bed awake by arising at a consistent morning time and staying up until a prescribed time in the evening, which is significantly later than usual. Time in bed is gradually expanded as sleep efficiency (total sleep time divided by the total time in bed) increases. Cognitive restructuring is the last active CBT-I component. It is a cognitive intervention in which practitioners use guided discovery to help patients identify and change illogical or extreme ways of thinking.[17] In the context of sleep, these thoughts often relate to frustration over the inability to fall asleep or exaggerated concerns about the effects of sleep loss on daily functioning.[18]

Because insomnia is a predictor of depression recurrence, researchers have questioned whether CBT-I might have a valuable role as an adjunct treatment of depression. For instance, Manber and colleagues[19] assessed the impact of CBT-I in 30 individuals with depression and insomnia who were receiving concomitant treatment by escitalopram. Individuals were randomized to 7 weeks of individual CBT-I or an attention control condition using a validated quasidesensitization technique. Those individuals who received CBT-I had a higher rate of depression remission (61.5%) and insomnia remission (50.0%) than those who received the control condition (33.3% depression, 7.7% control), although these differences were not statistically significant (potentially because of the small sample size). These findings are consistent with a recent randomized control trial in which brief behavioral therapy for insomnia, a variant of CBT-I that does not use cognitive restructuring, and treatment as usual (controlled prescription of antidepressant) were compared with treatment as usual alone in patients with both refractory depression and insomnia.[20] Relative to treatment as usual alone, patients who received brief behavioral therapy for insomnia had significantly improved sleep quality and depression. In addition, 50% of patients receiving brief behavioral therapy for insomnia achieved depression remission after 8 weeks compared with only 5.9% of patients who did not receive the therapy. In total, these studies support the concept that augmentation of an antidepressant medication with CBT-I may not only improve insomnia but also depression outcomes.

Several studies have shown that CBT-I seems to be just as effective for insomnia in the context of comorbid depression as in patients without comorbid depression.[21–28] In one of the largest studies, Manber and colleagues[21] delivered seven sessions of group CBT-I to 301 patients referred for insomnia. They found no differences between individuals with higher versus lower levels of depression on sleep diary indices, insomnia severity, and well-being outcomes, demonstrating that depression is not contraindicated for CBT-I. In addition, the group of individuals with higher levels of depression experienced a significant reduction in depression symptoms and suicidal ideation from pre– to post–CBT-I. Depression severity dropped by at least one standard deviation (approximately seven points on the beck depression inventory [BDI]) indicating that this change was also clinically significant. Of note, only individuals who completed treatment were included in study analyses. Previous reports indicate that depression may predict drop-out of group CBT-I. Using receiver operating characteristic curve analyses, Ong and colleagues[29] found that 22% of patients with elevated depression symptom scores and at least 3.65 hours of sleep were early dropouts compared with 4.3% of those who reported fewer depression symptoms. Regardless of depression symptoms, individuals with reduced total sleep time (<3.65 hours of sleep) were at greatest risk for an early termination of CBT-I.

In general, depressed patients have more difficulties adhering to a fixed rise time, restricting time in bed, and changing expectations about sleep than individuals with less depression.[21] Behavioral interventions may be more challenging for depressed patients because of motivational deficits. Also, depressed patients may spend excessive time awake in bed in attempts to avoid daily demands, activities, or interactions with others. For similar reasons, individuals with depression may avoid arising early in the morning. Depressed individuals display attention biases to negative stimuli, which might render concern about next day consequences of poor sleep more salient. Therapists might find cognitive restructuring a larger undertaking in depressed individuals because automatic cognitive distortions are likely to be used frequently during the day and not limited specifically to sleep.

Given these factors, it is recommended that providers who use CBT-I in depressed patients attend to depression-related factors that could hinder adherence. For instance, providers might encourage depressed patients to plan positive activities in the morning that increase motivation to arise from bed.[21] They might also use behavioral activation principles by encouraging depressed patients to engage in activities that provide pleasure or mastery when feeling sad during the day, rather than retiring to the bed. Finally, it is recommended that CBT-I providers treating depressed patients expand use of cognitive interventions from sleep-specific cognitive distortions to address cognitive distortions that might lead to therapy nonadherence in general.

In summary, CBT-I is a well-tested evidenced-based therapy for insomnia that also seems to significantly reduce depression symptoms. Two studies have indicated that it augments antidepressant response. Depressed patients do not seem to have worse symptom outcomes than nondepressed patients. However, depressed patients may have some difficulties adhering to or finishing the therapy protocol. As such, it is recommended that CBT-I therapists incorporate elements of CBT-D into the therapy to address adherence problems caused by motivational deficits, avoidance, and depressogenic automatic thoughts.

COGNITIVE BEHAVIORAL THERAPY FOR DEPRESSION AND INSOMNIA

CBT-D is a well-tested, evidence-based therapy for depression that can be administered in group or individual format across 12 to 24 sessions. It is as effective as antidepressants for all severity levels of depression,[30] and it may be superior to antidepressants in preventing depression relapse.[31] The primary mechanisms for CBT-D are cognitive restructuring and behavioral activation. In cognitive therapy, patients are encouraged to recognize unhelpful thinking patterns, test their validity, and substitute more logical and helpful thoughts in their place. To test the validity of thoughts, patients must expose themselves to new situations or new patterns of behavior. This part of therapy encourages behavioral activation, which may actually be the most active ingredient of CBT-D.[32] In CBT-D, the therapist uses such techniques as Socratic questioning, role playing, imagery, guided discovery, assertiveness training, and behavioral experiments. CBT-D may also include elements of CBT-I, including stimulus control and relaxation therapy, and it may address sleep-relevant cognitions, although it is unclear how much this is used in actual CBT-D practice. CBT-D is structured, goal-oriented, and characterized by a collaborative therapeutic relationship that focuses on the present.

No studies to our knowledge have examined whether insomnia moderates response to CBT-D. In a prospective case-control study of 90 patients receiving cognitive therapy for depression, approximately 30% of individuals with abnormal architecture sleep profiles failed treatment versus 12% of individuals with normal sleep profiles.[33] The abnormal sleep group also had a significantly slower onset of remission. Sleep did not predict relapse, but abnormal sleepers had a lower rate of recovery and a higher rate of recurrence than normal sleepers. Further research in this area is clearly necessary.

Does CBT-D address insomnia symptoms? Carney and colleagues[34] found than approximately one-half of individuals with baseline sleep problems no longer experienced the relative sleep symptom after successful CBT-D. However, they noted that 50% of all successful CBT-D study patients experienced some form of insomnia symptom as a residual symptom (13% experienced early insomnia, 14% middle insomnia, and 8% late insomnia). These rates were lower than those reported by Taylor and colleagues[35] who found that 17%, 36%, and 24% of depressed patients who responded to cognitive therapy continued to experience early, middle, and late insomnia, respectively. They also found that 29% of responders continued to experience depressed mood and even more people continue to experience residual anxiety (37% experience psychological anxiety and 42% somatic anxiety). Moreover, insomnia was not a predictor of relapse/recurrence over 2 years follow-up when other factors, such as psychological anxiety, were included in the model.

Both of these studies analyzed sleep response using a global interview question for depression (Hamilton Depression Rating Scale). One study to date has examined pretherapy and posttherapy sleep changes using sleep diaries, the preferred assessment for insomnia.[36] Manber and colleagues[37] examined sleep diaries before and after 16 to 20 sessions of cognitive behavioral analysis system of psychotherapy, a version of CBT used in chronic depression that focuses on the interpersonal domain. The researchers found significant improvements in sleep efficiency, wake time after sleep onset, sleep onset latency, total sleep time, and early morning awakenings from baseline to the end of treatment. However, only 33% of patients who reported difficulties with early morning awakenings, 43% of patients with sleep maintenance difficulties, and 37% of patients with sleep-onset difficulties had a clinically significant improvement in sleep after cognitive behavioral analysis system of psychotherapy. These data concur with those reported by previous studies suggesting that insomnia is addressed by CBT-D but not as fully as it is with CBT-I.

One study to date has analyzed electroencephalographic variables before and after administration of CBT-D.[38] Consistent with insomnia findings, CBT-D was associated with an increase in sleep efficiency. Reduced rapid eye movement latency and reduced slow wave sleep (two sleep indices characteristic of depression) were stable across the course of therapy. The authors hypothesized that these variables are stable, trait-like phenomena of depression. No studies to our knowledge have examined whether individuals with insomnia are less adherent to CBT-D. Research has shown that sleep-deprived individuals have difficulties with sustained attention[39] and often choose to engage in less effortful versus more effortful tasks, if given the choice.[40] Theoretically, sleep-deprived individuals might be less adherent to CBT-D because of fatigue, avoidance, or difficulties with sustained attention that might lead to problems remembering how to implement skills. In particular, cognitive restructuring may be a complicated and effortful process for tired individuals.[13] Because insomnia does not equate to sleep deprivation, it is unclear how or if these findings relate to patients with insomnia. Nevertheless, this topic merits clinical investigation.

In summary, CBT-D is a well-tested evidenced-based therapy for depression that also seems to significantly reduce insomnia symptoms. Unfortunately, insomnia is a common residual symptom after CBT-D. One study suggested that residual insomnia after CBT-D did not predict relapse/recurrence above and beyond the impact of residual anxiety. Studies are necessary to examine whether insomnia moderates CBT-D treatment adherence or response. One study found that individuals with an abnormal electroencephalographic profile have worse CBT-D outcomes.

Researchers have suggested modifications to CBT-I with comorbid depression[21] and CBT-D with comorbid insomnia.[17] However, few studies to date have developed and tested a CBT that addresses both conditions. This might be beneficial to patients, given the ways that these disorders interact in perpetuating a negative clinical state. Next we review one such therapy we are currently developing and testing for patients with insomnia, depression, and posttraumatic stress disorder (PTSD): cognitive behavioral social rhythm therapy (CBSRT).

THERAPEUTIC OPTION: COGNITIVE BEHAVIORAL SOCIAL RHYTHM GROUP THERAPY FOR SLEEP DISTURBANCE, DEPRESSION, AND POSTTRAUMATIC STRESS DISORDER

CBSRT is based on the social rhythm model of mood disruption, in which it is hypothesized that a stressful life event interrupts a person's daily routine (social rhythms). This disruption then leads to instability in biologic rhythms and disrupted sleep in vulnerable individuals.[41] CBSRT is designed to improve mood and sleep by stabilizing social rhythms, increasing exposure to ambient light, changing dysfunctional bed/bedtime associations, and challenging dysfunctional automatic thoughts that might contribute to behavioral inactivation and nonadherence to the therapy protocol.

CBSRT is a 12-week, manualized CBT administered in a group format. CBSRT was designed as a skills group for a severe, comorbid Veterans Affairs population. Throughout treatment, metaphors are used to facilitate activation of the imagery system. Also, discussion of traumatic events is minimized; individuals are taught how to encounter present-day stressors that may interfere with current mood and daily routine. **Table 1** provides a description of the intervention.

To our knowledge, CBSRT is one of the first psychotherapies designed for veterans with insomnia and depression. Because depression onset is so often associated with a stressful life event, CBSRT may be readily applied to depressed individuals without PTSD. It addresses elements of depression, including behavioral inactivation, lack of motivation, and inconsistent or inactive daily routine that might interfere with implementation of stimulus control or sleep restriction. Cognitive restructuring is used early-on and more broadly than CBT-I to address cognitive distortions that patients might experience during the day and at night. Next is an example of a therapeutic exchange that demonstrates one way a CBSRT therapist might address a type of depressogenic cognitive distortion (emotional reasoning) that contributes to therapy nonadherence.

Therapist: I notice that you woke-up at 7 AM but did not get out of bed as we discussed. What do you think stood in the way?

Patient: I don't know. I am just overwhelmed and tired.

T: When you did get up for the day around 9 AM, did you feel any less overwhelmed or tired?

P: No. In fact, I felt worse for wasting that time and not getting out of bed like I should have.

T: So, what you're saying is that when you feel tired and overwhelmed and stay in bed, you feel even worse.

P: Correct

T: I'm wondering how you might feel if you changed that habit and got out of bed, even if you don't really feel like it?

Table 1	
Description of cognitive behavioral social rhythm therapy	
Models	Social rhythm theory of mood disturbance Behavioral activation Cognitive theory
Duration	12 wk, once per week 2 h: first hour, homework review; second hour, new material
Modality	Group therapy, manualized
Session 1–4	Patients are oriented to the cognitive behavioral model and taught thought-challenging skills. They begin monitoring their mood, thoughts, and daily habitual behaviors (or social rhythms).
Session 5–7	Patients create a daily routine. They are taught to use positive rewards and behavioral activation as a way of overcoming obstacles that might prevent them from adhering to their daily routine. Adherence issues are addressed with in-session cognitive restructuring practice.
Session 8–10	Session content transitions to a focus on sleep, including an introduction to stimulus control and imagery rehearsal for nightmares. Adherence issues are addressed with in-session cognitive restructuring practice.
Session 11–12	The final two sessions focus on relapse prevention and a summary of skills that they have learned.

P: I'm not sure.

T: Me neither. Would you be open to testing it out this week by getting out of bed?

P: I guess so. I have nothing to lose – I'm already feeling miserable.

In this example, the therapist identified ways that poor mood and anergia result from behavioral inactivity in the patient's current behavioral pattern. The therapist incorporated thought-challenging techniques commonly used in CBT-D to highlight this negative cycle and also encouraged the patient to engage an experiment to test whether he might feel less anergic if he were to change his behavior.

CLINICAL OUTCOMES

Analyses from a randomized controlled trial comparing CBSRT with present centered therapy (a Yalom-based process group) are pending. Open trial, intent-to-treat results are currently under review, but preliminary results indicate that 24 male veterans enrolled in CBSRT had significant improvements in sleep, anxiety, and depression symptoms,[42] although the clinical significance of depression symptom reduction was questionable.[42] The failure to observe a large reduction in depression symptoms is consistent with other studies showing an increased likelihood of treatment-resistant depression in comorbid anxiety.[43] Also, Vietnam War era veterans with PTSD have overall worse outcomes to psychotherapy[44] especially in a group format.[45]

Secondary analyses from the open trial demonstrated that veterans enrolled in CBSRT also had significant improvements in mood regulation,[46] as assessed by the Negative Mood Regulation questionnaire. Improvements in sleep diary parameters were not temporally related to improvements in mood regulation, but improvements in sleep perception (nightmare distress, sleep quality, and less morning sleepiness) were reciprocally related to mood regulation.[46] Thus, CBSRT seems to improve mood regulation abilities via mechanisms other than sleep improvement.

Cloitre and colleagues[47] studied women with PTSD from childhood sexual abuse. They found that higher pretreatment Negative Mood Regulation scores were associated with better response to PTSD exposure therapy. Thus, in the context of PTSD/major depressive disorder/insomnia morbidity, CBSRT may be best conceptualized as a Phase 1 approach to facilitate Phase 2 PTSD psychotherapy outcomes. CBSRT may also be a short-term group treatment administered to individuals who might be otherwise contraindicated to PTSD exposure therapies (eg, active/chronic suicidal ideation or recent/frequent psychiatric hospitalization). Future studies are necessary to test the efficacy of CBSRT in a community population of depressed individuals and also in depressed individuals without PTSD.

In summary, depression and insomnia are highly comorbid diagnostic states. CBT is an efficacious psychotherapy for insomnia and depression that involves change in behavioral habits, cognitive restructuring, and a collaborative therapeutic relationship characterized by guided discovery and neutral empiricism. Only a few studies have examined depression outcomes after CBT-I and insomnia outcomes after CBT-D. In general, CBT for each disorder seems to treat the alternate

disorder as well, although symptoms of the alternate disorder may remain in a significant number of individuals. Further research is necessary to test whether insomnia/depression comorbidity moderates therapy outcome and attrition. One study has found that depressed individuals may be less adherent to CBT-I, indicating a need to modify each therapy or implement a combined CBT approach for these individuals. CBSRT offers one such example of a combined approach, especially as part of a sequential treatment program in veterans with severe sleep disturbance, depression, and anxiety symptoms.

REFERENCES

1. Ohayon MM. Epidemiology of insomnia: what we know and what we still need to learn. Sleep Med Rev 2002;6:97–111.
2. American Psychiatric Association. Diagnostic and statistical manual of mental disorders. 5th edition. Arlington (VA): American Psychiatric Publishing; 2013.
3. Breslau N, Roth T, Rosenthal L, et al. Sleep disturbance and psychiatric disorders: a longitudinal epidemiological study of young adults. Biol Psychiatry 1996;39:411–8.
4. Ohayon MM, Roth T. Place of chronic insomnia in the course of depressive and anxiety disorders. J Psychiatr Res 2003;37:9–15.
5. Ford DE, Kamerow DB. Epidemiologic study of sleep disturbances and psychiatric disorders: an opportunity for prevention? JAMA 1989;262:1479–84.
6. Perlis ML, Giles DE, Buysee DJ, et al. Self-reported sleep disturbance as a prodormal symptom in recurrent depression. J Affect Disord 1997;42:209–12.
7. Schutte-Rodin S, Broch L, Buysse D, et al. Clinical guideline for the evaluation and management of chronic insomnia in adults. J Clin Sleep Med 2008; 4:487–504.
8. Buysse DJ, Angst J, Gamma A, et al. Prevalence, course, and comorbidity of insomnia and depression in young adults. Sleep 2008;31:473–80.
9. Kohn L, Espie CA. Sensitivity and specificity of measures of the insomnia experience: a comparative study of psychophysiologic insomnia, insomnia associated with mental disorder and good sleepers. Sleep 2005;28:104–12.
10. Carney CE, Edinger JD, Manber R, et al. Beliefs about sleep in disorders characterized by sleep and mood disturbance. J Psychosom Res 2007;62:179–88.
11. Kennedy GJ, Kelman HR, Thomas C. Persistence and remission of depressive symptoms in late life. Am J Psychiatry 1991;148:174–8.
12. Fawcett J, Scheftner WA, Fogg L, et al. Time-related predictors of suicide in major affective disorder. Am J Psychiatry 1990;147:1189–94.

13. Haynes PL, Ancoli-Israel S, Walter CM, et al. Preliminary evidence for a relationship between sleep disturbance and global attributional style in depression. Cognit Ther Res 2012;36:140–8.

14. Thase ME, Howland RH. Biological processes in depression: an updated review and integration. In: Beckham EE, Leber WR, editors. Biological processes in depression: an updated review and integration In: Handbook of Depression. 2nd Edition. New York: Guilford Press; 1995. p. 213–79.

15. Bootzin RR, Epstein D, Wood JM. Stimulus control instructions. In: Hauri P, editor. Case studies in insomnia. New York: Plenum Press; 1991. p. 19–28.

16. Spielman AJ, Saskin P, Thorpy MJ. Treatment of chronic insomnia by restriction of time in bed. Sleep 1987;10:45–56.

17. Beck AT, Rush AJ, Shaw BF, et al. Cognitive therapy of depression. New York: Guilford Press; 1979.

18. Morin C. Insomnia: psychological assessment and management. New York: Guilford Press; 1993.

19. Manber R, Edinger JD, Gress JL, et al. Cognitive behavioral therapy for insomnia enhances depression outcome in patients with comorbid major depressive disorder and insomnia. Sleep 2008;31:489–95.

20. Watanabe N, Furukawa TA, Shimodera S, et al. Brief behavioral therapy for refractory insomnia in residual depression: an assessor-blind, randomized controlled trial. J Clin Psychiatry 2011;72:1651–8.

21. Manber R, Bernert RA, Suh S, et al. CBT for insomnia in patients with high and low depressive symptom severity: adherence and clinical outcomes. J Clin Sleep Med 2011;7:645–52.

22. Edinger JD, Olsen MK, Stechuchak KM, et al. Cognitive behavioral therapy for patients with primary insomnia or insomnia associated predominantly with mixed psychiatric disorders: a randomized clinical trial. Sleep 2009;32:499–510.

23. Lichstein KL, Wilson NM, Johnson CT. Psychological treatment of secondary insomnia. Psychol Aging 2000;15:232–40.

24. Perlis ML, Sharpe M, Smith MT, et al. Behavioral treatment of insomnia: treatment outcome and the relevance of medical and psychiatric morbidity. J Behav Med 2001;24:281–96.

25. Taylor DJ, Lichstein KL, Weinstock J, et al. A pilot study of cognitive-behavioral therapy of insomnia in people with mild depression. Behav Ther 2007;38:49–57.

26. Hamoen AB, Redlich EM, de Weerd AW. Effectiveness of cognitive behavioral therapy for insomnia: influence of slight-to-moderate depressive symptom severity and worrying. Depress Anxiety 2014;31(8):662–8.

27. Thorndike FP, Ritterband LM, Gonder-Frederick LA, et al. A randomized controlled trial of an internet intervention for adults with insomnia: effects on comorbid psychological and fatigue symptoms. J Clin Psychol 2013;69:1078–93.

28. Lancee J, van den Bout J, van Straten A, et al. Baseline depression levels do not affect efficacy of cognitive-behavioral self-help treatment for insomnia. Depress Anxiety 2013;30:149–56.

29. Ong JC, Kuo TF, Manber R. Who is at risk for dropout from group cognitive-behavior therapy for insomnia? J Psychosom Res 2008;64:419–25.

30. DeRubeis RJ, Gelfand LA, Tang TZ, et al. Medications versus cognitive behavior therapy for severely depressed outpatients: mega-analysis of four randomized comparisons. Am J Psychiatry 1999;156:1007–13.

31. Hollon SD, DeRubeis RJ, Shelton RC, et al. Prevention of relapse following cognitive therapy vs medications in moderate to severe depression. Arch Gen Psychiatry 2005;62:417–22.

32. Jacobson NS, Dobson KS, Truax PA, et al. A component analysis of cognitive-behavioral treatment for depression. J Consult Clin Psychol 1996; 64:295–304.

33. Thase ME, Simons AD, Reynolds CF 3rd. Abnormal electroencephalographic sleep profiles in major depression: association with response to cognitive behavior therapy. Arch Gen Psychiatry 1996;53:99–108.

34. Carney CE, Segal ZV, Edinger JD, et al. A comparison of rates of residual insomnia symptoms following pharmacotherapy or cognitive-behavioral therapy for major depressive disorder. J Clin Psychiatry 2007;68:254–60.

35. Taylor DJ, Walters HM, Vittengl JR, et al. Which depressive symptoms remain after response to cognitive therapy of depression and predict relapse and recurrence? J Affect Disord 2010;123:181–7.

36. Buysse DJ, Ancoli-Israel S, Edinger JD, et al. Recommendations for a standard research assessment of insomnia. Sleep 2006;29:1155–73.

37. Manber R, Rush AJ, Thase ME, et al. The effects of psychotherapy, nefazodone, and their combination on subjective assessment of disturbed sleep in chronic depression. Sleep 2003;26:130–6.

38. Thase ME, Fasiczka AL, Berman SR, et al. Electroencephalographic sleep profiles before and after cognitive behavior therapy of depression. Arch Gen Psychiatry 1998;55:138–44.

39. Banks S, Dinges DF. Chronic sleep deprivation. In: Kryger MH, Roth T, Dement WC, editors. Principles and Practice of Sleep Medicine. 5th Edition. Philadelphia: Elsevier Saunders; 2011. p. 67–75.

40. Engle-Friedman M, Riela S, Golan R, et al. The effect of sleep loss on next day effort. J Sleep Res 2003; 12:113–24.

41. Ehlers CL, Frank E, Kupfer DJ. Social zeitgebers and biological rhythms. A unified approach to understanding the etiology of depression. Arch Gen Psychiatry 1988;45:948–52.

42. Haynes PL, Kelly M, Scheller V, et al. Stabilizing sleep and daily routine in veterans with comorbid PTSD and depression: follow-up outcomes for cognitive

behavioral social rhythm therapy. Sleep 2009; 32(Abstract Supplement):A344.

43. Sharma V, Mazmanian D, Persad E, et al. A comparison of comorbid patterns in treatment-resistant unipolar and bipolar depression. Can J Psychiatry 1995;40:270–4.

44. Bisson JI, Ehlers A, Matthews R, et al. Psychological treatments for chronic post-traumatic stress disorder. Systematic review and meta-analysis. Br J Psychiatry 2007;190:97–104.

45. Foa EB, Keane TM, Friedman MJ, et al, editors. Effective treatments for PTSD: practice guidelines

from the International Society for Traumatic Stress. New York: The Guilford Press; 2009.

46. Haynes PL, Kelly MR, Quan SF, et al. Cognitive behavioral social rhythm therapy is associated with significant improvement in capacity to regulate negative mood. Sleep 2010;33(Abstract Suppl): A247–8.

47. Cloitre M, Stovall-McClough KC, Miranda R, et al. Therapeutic alliance, negative mood regulation, and treatment outcome in child abuse-related post-traumatic stress disorder. J Consult Clin Psychol 2004;72:411–6.

Hypnosis in the Management of Sleep Disorders

Philip M. Becker, MD

KEYWORDS

- Hypnosis • Sleep disorders • Relaxation

KEY POINTS

- Although sleep and hypnosis share the same Greek root, they are distinct states of consciousness.
- Hypnosis offers potential therapeutic benefit for patients with sleep disorders, although the strength of evidenced-based therapy with hypnosis remains low.
- Hypnosis seems to benefit patients with primary insomnia, secondary insomnia comorbid with perimenopausal hot flashes or posttraumatic stress disorder, somnambulism, pavor nocturnus (sleep terrors), and sleep-related enuresis.
- Systematic study has generally been to a lesser standard then more common therapies of sleep disorders, primarily because of the difficulties of an adequate control condition.
- For professionals who receive training in hypnosis, there can be significant therapeutic value in understanding the language of change, patient receptivity to suggestion, and the potential contribution of hypnosis for patients with sleep disorders.

Hypnosis has been used to manage insomnia and disorders of arousal. Although hypnosis includes the Greek root word for sleep, the alteration in the state of consciousness that is produced during hypnotic trance is more similar to relaxed reverie than sleep. The electroencephalogram of hypnosis shows none of the slowing of the electroencephalograph typical to sleep onset, although slow rolling eye movements are common in association with visualization during a hypnotic state. Hypnosis typically occurs in a state of repose and the accomplished subject may have no recollection of the experience during a trance, 2 commonalities with sleep. Because hypnosis allows for relaxation, increased suggestibility, posthypnotic suggestion, imagery rehearsal, access to pre-conscious cognitions and emotions, and cognitive restructuring, disorders of sleep such as the insomnias, parasomnias, and related mood or anxiety disorders can be amenable to therapeutic intervention through hypnosis or training in self-hypnosis.

Hypnosis is best considered a therapeutic modality rather than a therapy in its own right. It should be offered within the context of a complete psychological and medical treatment plan and offers the advantage to facilitate sensations, perceptions, thoughts, feelings, or behaviors. In a review of the literature in 2008, researchers in Singapore described how hypnosis has been offered as treatment for acute and chronic insomnia, nightmares, sleep terrors, and other parasomnias such as head or body rocking, bedwetting, and sleepwalking. The authors point out that it is a challenge "to perform a randomized, double-blind, controlled trial to evaluate hypnotherapy given that cooperation and rapport between patient and therapist is needed to achieve a receptive trance state."[1]

Department of Psychiatry, Sleep Medicine Associates of Texas, University of Texas Southwestern Medical Center at Dallas, 5477 Glen Lakes Drive, Suite 100, Dallas, TX 75231, USA
E-mail address: pbecker@sleepmed.com

Sleep Med Clin 10 (2015) 85–92
http://dx.doi.org/10.1016/j.jsmc.2014.11.003
1556-407X/15/$ – see front matter © 2015 Elsevier Inc. All rights reserved.

THE MYTHS OF HYPNOSIS

Hypnosis is misunderstood by professionals and patients alike. Hypnosis is not mind control, simple suggestion, or gullibility. If you have a talent for hypnosis, it does not mean that you have a weak mind. At the same time that the Sleep Disorders Center at Stanford University was established, the University's Department of Psychology had a world-renowned researcher, Ernest Hilgard, investigating hypnotic phenomena such as his concept of the hidden observer.[2] The University of Pennsylvania was another reputable institution where hypnosis was studied. Catechol-O-methyltransferase polymorphism seems to be associated with the ability to enter a hypnotic trance on formal testing on a scale that is used to segment research subjects into groups of high and low hypnotizability.[3] Patients with sleep disorders may benefit because of the unique characteristics that hypnosis produces in relaxation and mental ease, absorption, orientation and monitoring, and self-agency. A challenge for this review is the primary method of report, case series, which lack significant experimental rigor, primarily because clinicians have offered description, and researchers in sleep medicine have generally not explored the use of hypnosis as a therapeutic modality.

HYPNOTIC INDUCTION/TRANCE

Practitioners of hypnosis have developed their own vocabulary to discuss the alterations in the state of consciousness that represents hypnotic trance.[4] The literature of hypnosis describes certain techniques for induction, deepening, pacing/leading, and posthypnotic suggestion. The use of therapeutic language through training in hypnosis is a significant advantage for any health care professional. Preparing the subject for hypnosis is like any appropriate therapeutic process that involves the setting of therapeutic goals and heightening expectancy. A trusting relationship facilitates entrance into trance. Focusing attention and the usage of repetition ("watch the watch," stare at an object across the room, or the point of a pencil, etc) allows the subject to alter consciousness more easily. Those who are interested in learning hypnotic technique should take a training course offered by professional organizations such as the American Society of Clinical Hypnosis. To assist understanding, a scenario is included that describes a hypnotic procedure that has been offered to insomnia patients (**Table 1**).

NEUROBIOLOGY OF HYPNOSIS

The electroencephalographic recording of subjects in a hypnotic state has no similarity to any stages of sleep. Hypnosis is associated with significant modulation of connectivity and activity within the brain. One research group identified a neural network that was most prominent in frontal regions of the brain, depending on the depth of the hypnotic state, the type of mental content and emotional involvement.[5] Hypnotizability as measured by structured assessment does not seem to have a significant effect on electroencephalographic activity, but hypnotic depth correlated with increased left anterior hemispheric slowing and decreased central fast electroencephalographic activity.[6] In a study of subjects with high hypnotizability (HH), the theta1 and theta2 spectral power was higher than in subjects with low hypnotizability. Coherence between distributed brain regions was sharply elevated in HH subjects within the theta and alpha frequency bands. The coherence between frontal and posterior areas within the beta–gamma frequency ranges was higher in HH subjects. The results suggest that HH subjects are engaged in imaginal mental activity, whereas low hypnotizability subjects are mainly engaged in linguistic activity.[7] In another study, HH participants reliably experienced greater state dissociation and exhibited lower frontal–parietal phase synchrony in the alpha2 frequency band during hypnosis than low hypnotizability participants. These findings suggest that HH individuals exhibit a disruption of the frontal–parietal network that is only observable during hypnotic induction.[8]

Neuroimaging studies also support information processing differences in HH subjects. Various studies have assessed state changes through hypnotic suggestions of typical phenomena. In a study of posthypnotic suggestion for amnesia (PHA), the PHA group showed reduced memory for details of a movie that was hypnotically "forgotten" but not for the context of the viewing of the movie. Activity in occipital, temporal, and prefrontal areas differed among the control and PHA groups, and between the PHA group during hypnotic amnesia and reversal of amnesia. The study authors opine that the more activated regions interrupt retrieval of long-term episodic memory, inhibiting retrieval.[9] It has been proposed that the activation of a portion of the prefrontal cortex in response to both hypnotic suggestions for decreased pain and to positive emotional experience might indicate an underlying mechanism of hypnotizability.[10] Changes in relaxation, mental ease, and absorption during standard hypnotic procedures are associated with changes in brain activity within structures critically involved in the basic representation of the body–self and the regulation of states of consciousness, supporting

Table 1
Scenario: Example of one hypnotic technique for insomnia that would be offered to a patient who is ready to use hypnosis/self-hypnosis for sleep

Induction	Straighten your left arm in front of your eyes. Now bend the back of your hand up at the wrist. Concentrate on a spot in the back of your hand....
	Focus your eyes on that spot as you focus on the sound of my voice. In a little while you will feel your hand and arm getting heavy....
	As the hand and arm get heavy, you will notice how the hand and arm want to lower down to your leg....
	Your hand and arm are heavier and heavier. It's like a weight is pulling down on the arm. You are more and more ready to feel the relief of resting your hand down... (continue suggestions until down movement first starts, and then encourage it)
	Very good, you are doing very well. Now notice how your eyelids feel heavier and heavier as the weight pulls your hand down to rest on your leg or side....
	Very good. You are almost there. Your hand, your arm, your eyelids heavier and heavier. Your eyelids are ready to close. When your hand comes to rests, your eyelids will close....
	With your hand resting and your eyelids closed, you are now ready to experience deeper relaxation....
Deepening	Notice how heavy your hand and arm feel....
	Notice that the heaviness is getting a bit stronger each time you exhale....
	Breathe in and then feel the heaviness as you breathe out....
	That's right. Notice your breathing. Breathe out and the heaviness grows as your body relaxes....
	Are you ready to relax even more deeply so that you can sleep soundly and deeply? Of course, you are. Deep sleep is what you are here for....
	Notice how heavy your hand and arm feel....
	Now notice how your shoulder is getting heavy....
	That's right. The heaviness, the relaxation is spreading out of your arm and into your body....
	Your shoulder is heavy and relaxed. With each exhalation, the comfort, the relaxation spreads across your shoulders into your other arm and down your chest all the way to your back....
	Very good. Feel as it spreads through your body, down into your legs....
	As it spreads, feel how you are free of tension, free of tightness, free of stress, free of strain....
	A wonderful heaviness like being held in a wonderful embrace. Any tension or tightness or stress or strain flow out of you as you breathe out....
	That's right just breathe out any last tension, tightness, stress, strain as the comfortable relaxation begins to spread up into your face....
	Feel how relaxed and comfortable your mouth, cheeks, and eyelids, even your eyes themselves, forehead, and earlobes, even your scalp and tongue feel so relaxed....
	Now your mind is ready to fall into deep sleep.
Pacing/leading suggestions: the circle of deep sleep	Now check yourself to see if there is any last tension or tightness that needs to be blown out. Take a deep breath. Hold that breath. Collect the last little bit of tension and tightness. Now let the breath go, and feel the last of the tension and tightness flow out of you....
	Very good. Now deep, sound sleep....
	Imagine that you are in a wonderful and comfortable place. A place where you feel safe and secure. A place free of tension and tightness. A place free of stress and strain. You are deeply relaxed. You are at peace with your self and with the world. There is nothing more to do than enjoy deep sleep.
	Now it's time for you to receive important suggestions. Your body is ready. You are ready. Imagine a way to write without using a hand. This is writing with your mind....

(continued on next page)

Table 1 (continued)	
	Just let your mind decide what is best. Some imagine clouds forming the number and letters. Another sees sky writing. Some discover it is on a TV or computer. I personally like the magic blackboard. Just listen and see what happens as you are ready to receive deep sleep. Very good….
	Now draw a box and a circle. Watch the center of the box where your mind is writing 100. Right there, the number 100 appears. Notice how 100 is very slowly fading even as you move to the circle. Now in the circle, watch as your mind receives the next writing. Watch the circle expand and 100 disappear as the letters appear …D…E…E…P……S…L…E…E…P.
	You are creating deep sleep with every letter….
	As you watch the box, 99 begins to appear even as the circle of deep sleep is absorbed back into your mind. Now watch the circle as the letters return, …D…E…E…P……S…L…E…E…P.
	As you create each letter of deep sleep, the numbers in the box countdown and fade away. With the next number, 98, the circle of deep sleep is absorbed into your mind and grows deeper and deeper into your mind. …D…E…E…P……S…L…E…E…P
	Then 97, …D…E…E…P……S…L…E…E…P
	Then 96, …D…E…E…P……S…L…E…E…P
	On it goes as you absorb deep sleep.
Posthypnotic suggestion	Very good. You have done very well. And as you practice, you will do even better….
	You are almost ready to bring the box and circle to bed.
	You want and you need to make …D…E…E…P……S…L…E…E…P… a habit. A habit that becomes a wonderful part of you.
	Every day over the next week consider where and when you can practice your wonderful habit of deep sleep….
	Whether the morning, afternoon, or evening, take the time to make the wonderful habit of deep sleep your very own. See the number box and absorbing circle of deep sleep in normal activities.
	When brushing your teeth in morning and night, there is the circle of deep sleep. A stop sign reminds you to stop daydreaming and remember the circle of deep sleep. In your daily activities, there is the circle of deep sleep. The circle of deep sleep is a part of you as you pick up utensils to eat, relaxing with TV, the last chores, reading, sitting at the computer.
	It will be very interesting how the circle of deep sleep appears to you through the day. Watch and take pleasure in the circle of deep sleep.
	Now, see yourself walking into your bedroom to the circle of deep sleep. Preparing for bed and the circle surrounds you. The circle embracing you like your very first love….
	You are ready to welcome deep sleep. You can see yourself getting comfortable in bed.
	You raise your hand and arm about a foot off the bed. When heavy, it drifts down. The heaviness spreads across your chest, down your legs and up to your face even into your brain and mind. Without even thinking about it, 100 appears in the box. As 100 fades, the circle …D…E…E…P……S…L…E…E…P appears.
	As the circle of deep sleep is absorbed into your mind, 99 appears, then the next circle of deep sleep is absorbed, then 98 and the next circle as you fall into a comfortable, deep, refreshing sleep. If you wake up for the bathroom or any reason, the box and circle reappear and you start where you left off inside the circle of deep sleep. You may discover, like others have done before, that it is uncommon to remember a number beyond 95.
Deinduction	Very good. You have done very well. Deep sleep is more a part of you.
	I congratulate you on your success today and how well you will do tonight and most every night. I don't really know. There may be nights of disturbed sleep and that is just fine. Remember: accept any night of sleep, whether light or deep. Light nights help you to appreciate even more the nights of deep sleep.
	Now, I will bring you back to the room we are sitting in. I will count from 10 to 1. As I count, you will feel your mind becoming more and more alert. A wonderful feeling of relaxed awareness returns to your arms and legs and body.
	10 and 9, ready to enjoy all that you accomplished; 8 and 7, more alert; 6 and 5, the wonderful feeling of relaxed awareness returning to your arms and legs and body; 4, 3, 2, very good, almost there; 1 and aware of your body, the room, and what you have accomplished.

the view that hypnosis is an altered state of consciousness.[11] Although not specifically studied with hypnosis, there has been increasing interest in the precuneus region of the brain in chronic insomnia, a region that is associated with self-image. Primary insomnia patients who were studied had a smaller volume of gray matter in the left orbitofrontal cortex that strongly correlated ($r = -0.71$) with the subjective severity of insomnia as well as in the anterior and posterior precuneus. Patients did not show any other regional differences.[12] A Russian study of somatosensory evoked potentials in 2 patients who were implanted with multiple deep brain electrodes in preparation for treatment of their obsessive–compulsive disorder demonstrated in the 1 patient who was highly suggestible that there was involvement of the anterior cingulate cortex and the anterior temporal cortex in the control of pain during hypnotically suggested analgesia.[13]

HYPNOSIS AND INSOMNIA

Behavioral techniques such as hypnosis have a role in the management of insomnia. Earlier papers provide conceptualization or limited review of hypnosis for insomnia, often making insufficient definition of the hypnotic experience and other therapeutic modalities. A paper in 1982 described insomnia as a pervasive clinical problem that is amenable to therapy with hypnosis for secondary disorders such as depression, pain, anxiety, and lifestyle change being improved when combined with progressive relaxation and ego strengthening.[14] Twenty-five years later, there was a similar impression that there was little empirical research pertaining to the use of hypnotherapy as either a single treatment or multitreatment modality for the management of sleep disorders.[15] A National Institutes of Health Technology Assessment Panel on Integration of Behavioral and Relaxation Approaches into the Treatment of Chronic Pain and Insomnia concluded that behavioral techniques for insomnia, particularly relaxation and biofeedback that have similarity to hypnosis, produce improvements in some aspects of sleep, but it is questionable whether the magnitude of the improvement in sleep onset and total sleep time are clinically significant.[16]

In the hypnosis literature, there are case series that identify therapeutic improvement on insomnia with hypnosis. Forty-five subjects were matched on their baseline sleep onset latency by sleep diary and then randomly assigned to hypnotic relaxation, stimulus control and placebo. Each group received 4 weekly sessions of 30 minutes' duration. Hypnotic relaxation treatment was reported to be effective in reducing sleep onset latency. Neither stimulus control nor placebo groups recorded similar improvement.[17] In a retrospective case series with children, 75 pediatric patients (mean age, 12 years; range, 7–17) received a single relaxation session with hypnosis and then returned for follow-up. When insomnia did not resolve after the first hypnotic relaxation session, patients were offered the opportunity to use enhanced recall under hypnosis to gain insight into the cause of insomnia. Younger children were more likely to report that the insomnia was related to fears. Two or fewer hypnosis sessions were provided to 68% of the patients. In 70 patients reporting a delay in sleep onset latency of more than 30 minutes, 90% reported a reduction in sleep onset time after hypnosis. Of the 21 patients reporting nighttime awakenings more than once a week, 52% reported resolution of the awakenings and 38% reported improvement. A subanalysis of 29 patients was undertaken with subjective somatic complaints, such as chest pain, dyspnea, functional abdominal pain, habit cough, headaches, and vocal cord dysfunction; 87% reported improvement or resolution of the somatic complaints after hypnosis.[18] In another study at a sleep disorders center, 13 patients with persistent psychophysiologic insomnia received evaluation for chronic primary insomnia that occurred on at least 3 nights per week for 6 months or longer. Six patients accepted hypnotherapy that was conducted in 1 to 3 sessions (mean, 1.7). Three patients responded to 2 sessions of hypnotherapy that included a relaxation exercise and the image of the blackboard where they counted down from 100 and wrote the suggestion "deep sleep." The 3 responders remained improved at 16-month follow-up. Factors that seemed to contribute to long-term response in this small group of patients included a report of sleeping at least half of the time while in bed (sleep efficiency >50%), increased hypnotic susceptibility, no history of major depression, and a lack of secondary gain.[19]

Use of Hypnosis for Insomnia Comorbid with Other Disorders

Hot flashes are a significant problem for many breast cancer survivors and can cause discomfort, insomnia, anxiety, and decreased quality of life. Menopausal women also seek nonpharmacologic treatment. In a study of hypnotic treatment of hot flashes and fatigue, 10 healthy postmenopausal women and 4 breast cancer patients were treated with 4, weekly sessions of 1 hour of hypnosis by the same physician and nurse. Daily frequency, duration, and severity were recorded on a hot flashes diary. Quality of life and fatigue were recorded by the Quality of Life Questionnaire-Core 36 (QLQ-C30) and Brief Fatigue Inventory. The frequency ($P<.0001$), duration ($P<.0001$), and severity ($P<.0001$) of hot flashes were significantly reduced. The overall quality of life was also improved ($P = .05$). The subjects enjoyed better sleep and had less insomnia ($P = .012$). There was a significant improvement in current fatigue level ($P = .017$), but there was no reduction in the total fatigue level.[20] In a literature review of hypnosis to reduce hot flashes, hypnosis was considered to be of significant benefit in treatment of hot flashes while also reducing anxiety and improving sleep. It seems to be associated with few side effects and was preferred by women who wish to forego hormonal therapy.[21]

In an Israeli study that compared adjunctive hypnotherapy and zolpidem in patients with insomnia and chronic posttraumatic stress disorder, 32 patients with posttraumatic stress disorder who were already treated with selective serotonin reuptake inhibitors (antidepressants) and supportive psychotherapy were randomized to 2 groups. Group 1 had 15 patients who took zolpidem 10 mg nightly for 2 weeks. Group 2 included 17 patients who received symptom-oriented hypnotherapy, twice weekly in 1.5-hour sessions over 2 weeks. All patients completed the Stanford Hypnotic Susceptibility Scale-Form C, Beck Depression Inventory, Impact of Event Scale, and Visual Subjective Sleep Quality Questionnaire before and after treatment. There was a significant main effect of the hypnotherapy treatment with posttraumatic stress disorder symptoms as measured by the Posttraumatic Disorder Scale. This effect was preserved at follow-up 1 month later. Additional benefits for the hypnotherapy group were decreases in intrusive thoughts/images and avoidance reactions as well as improvement in all assessed sleep variables.[22]

HYPNOSIS AND PARASOMNIAS

Hypnosis has also been used to improve disorders of arousal from sleep, including somnambulism (sleepwalking) and pavor nocturnus (sleep terrors). In general, reports of therapeutic benefit are limited to a small number of cases, case series, and a study of case controls. The first case series report was in 12 healthy service men facing honorable discharge from military service because of intractable sleepwalking. Six chose to participate in a short-term treatment program involving hypnosis. Four of the 6 young, male subjects reported total alleviation of symptoms.[23] The same

primary author pursued additional study with a single-blind, rater-blind, modified crossover design to evaluate a simple, practical method of clinical treatment of sleepwalking. Subjects had significant somnambulism without psychiatric illness and responded well to 6 brief sessions of symptom-focused hypnotherapy. Follow-up at 1 year demonstrated lasting improvement of both subjective and objective symptoms of sleepwalking. Hypnosis seems to reduce the sleep and emotional symptoms.[24]

Hurwitz and colleagues,[25] at a sleep disorder center that specializes in the management of parasomnias, studied the use of hypnosis as treatment for sleepwalking and sleep terror. Assessment was made of self-hypnotic treatment of 27 adult patients who chose hypnotic treatment in bed when falling off to sleep rather than pharmacotherapy. Using investigator-rated clinical global improvement, 74% of patients with clinically significant sleepwalking and/or sleep terrors showed much or very much improvement when followed over a number of months after their training in self-hypnosis. Training was brief, involving an average of 1.6 office visits. The authors conclude that hypnotic therapy represents a very cost-effective and noninvasive treatment modality, especially when contrasted with lengthy psychotherapy or long-term pharmacotherapy.[25] In a replication study of similar design completed at the Mayo Clinic Rochester, 36 patients were treated with self-hypnosis. The patients with parasomnias, mean age 32.7 years (range, 6–71), included 17 females and 4 children (age range, 6–16 years). The authors reported that all patients had chronic, "functionally autonomous" (self-sustaining) parasomnias that were treated in 1 or 2 hypnotherapy sessions. Therapeutic response was assessed by questionnaire over 5 years, demonstrating that 45.4% were symptom-free or at least much improved at the 1-month follow-up, 42.2% at the 18-month follow-up, and 40.5% at the 5-year follow-up.[26]

Another application for therapeutic hypnosis is sleep-related enuresis (bedwetting). When systematically reviewed, the efficacy of hypnosis and other behavioral interventions for sleep-related enuresis seems to be low based on evidenced-based criteria for rating.[27] The weakness of evidence is primarily because of the case series format with little consistency of control or assessment tools. Even with the reduced strength of the evidence, it seems that hypnosis may have a longer lasting effect than other therapeutic interventions for sleep-related enuresis. In a case-control study of hypnotherapy in the treatment of sleep-related enuresis on 48 boys, ages 8 to 13 years, subjects received 6 standardized sessions of 1 hour per week. The authors concluded that hypnotherapy was significantly effective over 6 months in decreasing enuretic episodes when compared with both pretreatment baseline enuresis frequency and no-treatment controls. Bringing into question whether the therapeutic response was related to hypnosis, the authors stated that "trance induction" was not required for success.[28] In a study from India, the efficacy of imipramine and hypnotic suggestions with imagery were compared for the management of functional nocturnal enuresis. Children (ages 5–16 years) with sleep-related enuresis underwent 3 months of therapy with imipramine (n = 25) or hypnosis (n = 25). The hypnosis group was instructed to continue practicing self-hypnosis daily during the 6-month follow-up period. Of the patients treated with imipramine, 76% had a positive response (all dry beds). In the patients treated with hypnotic suggestion with images of a dry bed, 72% remained dry over the night. At 9-month follow-up, 68% of patients in the hypnosis group maintained a positive response, whereas only 24% of the imipramine group remained fully dry. Hypnosis and self-hypnosis strategies were considered to be less effective in younger children (5–7 years old) compared with imipramine treatment. As reported in the previous study, the Indian authors reported that treatment response was not related to the "hypnotic responsivity" of the patient in either hypnosis or imipramine group.[29]

SUMMARY

Although sleep and hypnosis share the same Greek root, they are distinct states of consciousness. Hypnosis is still somewhat of a mystery regarding its psychophysiological, neuroanatomic, and behavioral manifestations. Hypnosis offers potential therapeutic benefit for patients with sleep disorders, although the strength of evidenced-based therapy with hypnosis remains low. In case series or case controls, hypnosis seems to provide benefit for patients with primary insomnia, secondary insomnia comorbid with perimenopausal hot flashes or posttraumatic stress disorder, somnambulism, pavor nocturnus (sleep terrors), and sleep-related enuresis. Systematic study has generally been to a lesser standard then more common therapies of sleep disorders, primarily because of the difficulties of an adequate control condition. Publications generally have come from clinicians rather than the research laboratory, also reducing the standard for evidence of therapeutic efficacy. Additional study is required to weight the relevance of suggestion, placebo effect, and the caring environment from the therapeutic benefit of "altered state" or "trance induction." For professionals who receive training in hypnosis, there can be significant therapeutic value in the understanding of language of change, patient receptivity to suggestion, and the potential unique contribution that hypnosis can have for patients with sleep disorders.

REFERENCES

1. Ng BY, Lee TS. Hypnotherapy for sleep disorders. Ann Acad Med Singapore 2008;37(8):683–8.
2. Hilgard E. Divided consciousness: multiple controls in human thought and action. New York: Wiley; 1977.
3. Szekely A, Kovacs-Nagy R, Bányai EI, et al. Association between hypnotizability and the catechol-O-methyltransferase (COMT) polymorphism. Int J Clin Exp Hypn 2010;58(3):301–15.
4. Hammond DC. Handbook of hypnotic suggestions and metaphor. New York: WW Norton and Company, Inc; 1990.
5. Lipari S, Baglio F, Griffanti L, et al. Altered and asymmetric default mode network activity in a "hypnotic virtuoso": an fMRI and EEG study. Conscious Cogn 2011;21(1):393–400.
6. Cardeña E, Lehmann D, Faber PL, et al. EEG sLORETA functional imaging during hypnotic arm levitation and voluntary arm lifting. Int J Clin Exp Hypn 2012;60(1):31–53.
7. Kirenskaya AV, Novototsky-Vlasov VY, Zvonikov VM. Waking EEG spectral power and coherence differences between high and low hypnotizable subjects. Int J Clin Exp Hypn 2011;59(4):441–53.
8. Terhune DB, Cardeña E, Lindgren M. Differential frontal-parietal phase synchrony during hypnosis as a function of hypnotic suggestibility. Psychophysiology 2011;48(10):1444–7.
9. Mendelsohn A, Chalamish Y, Solomonovich A, et al. Mesmerizing memories: brain substrates of episodic memory suppression in posthypnotic amnesia. Neuron 2008;57(1):159–70.
10. Feldman JB. The neurobiology of pain, affect and hypnosis. Am J Clin Hypn 2004;46(3):187–200.
11. Rainville P, Price DD. Hypnosis phenomenology and the neurobiology of consciousness. Int J Clin Exp Hypn 2003;51(2):105–29.
12. Altena E, Vrenken H, Van Der Werf YD, et al. Reduced orbitofrontal and parietal gray matter in chronic insomnia: a voxel-based morphometric study. Biol Psychiatry 2010;67(2):182–5.
13. Kropotov JD, Crawford HJ, Polyakov YI. Somatosensory event-related potential changes to painful stimuli during hypnotic analgesia: anterior cingulate cortex and anterior temporal cortex intracranial recordings. Int J Psychophysiol 1997;27(1):1–8.

14. Paterson DC. Hypnosis: an alternate approach to insomnia. Can Fam Physician 1982;28:768–70.

15. Graci GM, Hardie JC. Evidenced-based hypnotherapy for the management of sleep disorders. Int J Clin Exp Hypn 2007;55(3):288–302.

16. Integration of behavioral and relaxation approaches into the treatment of chronic pain and insomnia. NIH technology assessment panel on integration of behavioral and relaxation approaches into the treatment of chronic pain and insomnia. JAMA 1996;276(4):313–8.

17. Stanton HE. Hypnotic relaxation and the reduction of sleep onset insomnia. Int J Psychosom 1989;36(1–4):64–8.

18. Anbar RD, Slothower MP. Hypnosis for treatment of insomnia in school-age children: a retrospective chart review. BMC Pediatr 2006;6:23.

19. Becker PM. Chronic insomnia: outcome of hypnotherapeutic intervention in six cases. Am J Clin Hypn 1993;36(2):98–105.

20. Younus J, Simpson I, Collins A, et al. Mind control of menopause. Womens Health Issues 2003;13(2):74–8.

21. Elkins G, Marcus J, Palamara L, et al. Can hypnosis reduce hot flashes in breast cancer survivors? A literature review. Am J Clin Hypn 2004;47(1):29–42.

22. Abramowitz EG, Barak Y, Ben-Avi I, et al. Hypnotherapy in the treatment of chronic combat-related PTSD patients suffering from insomnia: a randomized, zolpidem-controlled clinical trial. Int J Clin Exp Hypn 2008;56(3):270–80.

23. Reid WH. Treatment of somnambulism in military trainees. Am J Psychother 1975;29(1):101–6.

24. Reid WH, Ahmed I, Levie CA. Treatment of sleepwalking: a controlled study. Am J Psychother 1981;35(1):27–37.

25. Hurwitz TD, Mahowald MW, Schenck CH, et al. A retrospective outcome study and review of hypnosis as treatment of adults with sleepwalking and sleep terror. J Nerv Ment Dis 1991;179(4):228–33.

26. Hauri PJ, Silber MH, Boeve BF. The treatment of parasomnias with hypnosis: a 5-year follow-up study. J Clin Sleep Med 2007;3(4):369–73.

27. Glazener CM, Evans JH, Cheuk DK. Complementary and miscellaneous interventions for nocturnal enuresis in children. Cochrane Database Syst Rev 2005;(2):CD005230.

28. Edwards SD, van der Spuy HI. Hypnotherapy as a treatment for enuresis. J Child Psychol Psychiatry 1985;26(1):161–70.

29. Banerjee S, Srivastav A, Palan BM. Hypnosis and self-hypnosis in the management of nocturnal enuresis: a comparative study with imipramine therapy. Am J Clin Hypn 1993;36(2):113–9.

Insomnia and Anxiety
Diagnostic and Management Implications of Complex Interactions

Robert N. Glidewell, PsyD, CBSM[a,b,*],
E. McPherson Botts, PsyD[c], William C. Orr, PhD[d]

KEYWORDS

• Anxiety • Insomnia • Sleep • Cognitive-behavior therapy • Epidemiology

KEY POINTS

• Mutual risk exists between anxiety and insomnia.
• Age-of-onset seems to be a prominent factor in the association between anxiety and insomnia, with early treatment of anxiety possibly reducing incident insomnia.
• Although anxiety is often temporally primary, conceptualization of insomnia and anxiety as comorbid and requiring independent diagnostic and therapeutic attention is warranted.
• Concurrent therapy for anxiety and insomnia is associated with improved sleep and augmented anxiolytic outcomes compared with monotherapies for anxiety.

INTRODUCTION

Insomnia and anxiety, respectively, are the most prevalent sleep and psychiatric disorders in the general adult population.[1,2] Forty percent to 92% of all cases of insomnia occur in the context of psychiatric disorders.[1,3] The prevalence of anxiety disorders in patients with insomnia is estimated to be 20% to 30%.[4] Given these facts, health care providers in all settings can expect these 2 conditions to present in a comorbid manner on a routine basis.

The relationship between insomnia and anxiety is increasingly recognized as complex and interactive. Although insomnia and anxiety are each associated with poorer health, increased health care utilization, daytime functional impairments, and generally poorer quality of life, they seem to have independent and additive deleterious effects when they cooccur.[5,6] Insomnia is an independent risk factor for incident anxiety disorders and vice versa.[1,3,7,8] The presence of insomnia differentially affects the course of individual anxiety disorders.[9] Accordingly, accurate diagnosis and management of comorbid insomnia and anxiety require a thorough understanding of their complex relationship.

With these issues in mind, the current article is intended to provide a focused review of the evidence on the relationship between insomnia and anxiety. Following a brief discussion of preliminary diagnostic and theoretic considerations, epidemiologic and treatment outcome research examining the insomnia-anxiety relationship is reviewed. Research on the specific subjective and objective manifestation of insomnia within specific anxiety disorders is not reviewed here.

Funding Sources: None.
Conflict of Interest: None.
[a] Insomnia Clinic, Behavioral Sleep Medicine, LLC, 315 East San Rafael Street, Colorado Springs, CO 80903, USA; [b] Department of Medicine, National Jewish Health, 1400 Jackson Street, Denver, CO 80206, USA; [c] Private Practice, 413 Security Boulevard, Suite C-5, Colorado Springs, CO 80911, USA; [d] Department of Physiology, University of Oklahoma Health Sciences Center, Lynn Health Science Institute, 3555 Northwest 58th Street, Suite 800, Oklahoma City, OK 73112, USA
* Corresponding author. Behavioral Sleep Medicine, LLC, 315 East San Rafael Street, Colorado Springs, CO 80903.
E-mail address: robert@sleeplivework.com

1556-407X/15/$ – see front matter © 2015 Elsevier Inc. All rights reserved.

PRELIMINARY CONSIDERATIONS
Putative Relationships Between Insomnia and Anxiety

In a recent update on the associations between anxiety and insomnia, Uhde and colleagues[10] proposed 2 primary models of the relationship. In the first model, anxiety and insomnia are each separate manifestations of an, as yet, undetermined core neurobiological diathesis. The brain responds to repeated challenges to the vulnerability or predisposition with the development of symptoms of anxiety and insomnia. In the second model, anxiety and insomnia are recognized as distinct disorders that either (1) each cause similar symptoms/morbidity over time or (2) are the consequence of another highly prevalent unspecified factor.

Comorbid Versus Secondary Insomnia

A growing body of evidence supports the need for a shift away from traditional conceptualizations of insomnia as a secondary symptom of medical and psychiatric disorders.[11] The National Institutes of Health held a State of the Science conference on the manifestation and management of chronic insomnia in adults in 2005. The final statement from this conference discouraged the term secondary insomnia in favor of the term comorbid insomnia.

Recommendation of the term comorbid insomnia was based on 2 primary concerns.[11] First, substantial concern was expressed that use of the term secondary insomnia was resulting in significant underdiagnosis and undertreatment of insomnia. Second, the term secondary insomnia implies an understanding of etiologic factors of insomnia that current evidence fails to provide. A substantial body of research supports the independent diagnosis of insomnia in the context of anxiety disorders specifically and psychiatric disorders generally. The remainder of this section reviews research on the relationship between insomnia and anxiety from epidemiologic and treatment perspectives.

INSOMNIA AND ANXIETY: BIDIRECTIONAL RISK

- Insomnia increases the risk for new onset anxiety disorders, and this risk increases with greater severity and chronicity of insomnia.
- Anxiety increases the risk for new onset insomnia diagnosis, and anxiety severity is related to insomnia severity.

Insomnia as a Risk Factor for Anxiety and Anxiety Disorders

Multiple longitudinal epidemiologic studies have examined the relationship between insomnia and anxiety disorders. Ford and Kamerow[3] analyzed the relationship between sleep disturbance and psychiatric disorders in 7954 subjects from the National Institutes of Mental Health Epidemiologic Catchment Area study. Subjects in this study were interviewed at baseline for the presence of sleep and psychiatric symptoms within the previous 6 months. A follow-up interview was completed 1 year later. At baseline, insomnia was present in 10% of subjects, and subjects with insomnia were more likely to have an anxiety disorder than subjects with no sleep complaint (23.9% vs 10%, $P<.001$).

Analysis of the 1-year follow-up data from the Ford and Kamerow study reveals insomnia to be a significant risk factor for anxiety disorders. **Fig. 1** shows the incidence of new anxiety disorders and the adjusted risk (odds ratio [OR]) for developing an anxiety disorder in subjects with insomnia at each time point as compared with

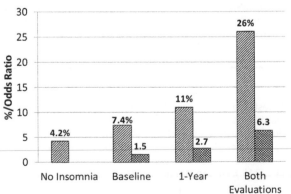

Fig. 1. Incidence and ORs for anxiety disorders in subjects with insomnia as compared with those with no sleep complaint. (*Data from* Ford DE, Karnerow DB. Epidemiologic study of sleep disturbances and psychiatric disorders. JAMA 1989;262:1479–84.)

individuals with no sleep complaint. As the figure shows, insomnia at any time point is associated with increased incidence and risk for development of an anxiety disorder. However, it is particularly important to note that subjects with insomnia at both time points experienced incident anxiety disorders at a rate 6 times greater than those subjects with no sleep complaint and 2 to 3 times greater than subjects reporting insomnia at a single time point. This finding strongly suggests that the chronic or episodic nature of insomnia is an important component of its relationship with anxiety.

Breslau and colleagues[1] have replicated and extended the above findings by examining lifetime prevalence and controlling for confounding psychiatric diagnostic and symptom factors. They examined these relationships in a 1200-person sample of 21-year-old to 30-year-old adults using the Diagnostic Interview Schedule–Revised. Subjects in this study were interviewed at baseline for lifetime history of sleep and psychiatric disorders. A follow-up interview for interval history of sleep and psychiatric disorders was completed 3.5 years later. In their sample, the lifetime prevalence of insomnia was 25% with 45% of those with insomnia at baseline also endorsing the presence of insomnia 3.5 years later. At baseline, anxiety disorders were significantly more prevalent in subjects with a history of insomnia compared with those without a history of insomnia (36% vs 19%, OR = 2.4). Based on the 3.5-year follow-up, incident anxiety disorders were also higher for subjects with insomnia (13.7% vs 7.1%, OR = 1.97). Similar findings were reported by 2 additional independent groups more recently.[7,8]

Although they did not perform a longitudinal study, Taylor and colleagues[12] further refined this line of investigation by using empirically validated insomnia criteria consistent with a diagnosis of chronic insomnia (previous studies required symptom duration of only 2 weeks) and controlling for major potential confounds, including medical illness and organic sleep disorders. In their community-based sample of 772 subjects aged 20 to 89 years old, subjects with insomnia were 17.35 times more likely than those without insomnia to have clinically significant anxiety. In addition, greater insomnia frequency was associated with increased severity of anxiety (t_{143} = 2.28, $P<.05$) but no other insomnia severity variables.

Anxiety and Anxiety Disorders as Risk Factors for Insomnia

At least 2 studies have examined the incidence of and risk for insomnia in patients with anxiety disorders. In a longitudinal population-based study of 2363 subjects, anxiety was found to be a significant risk factor for incident insomnia.[8] In this study, the incidence of insomnia over a period of 1 year was 14.6%. Compared with nonanxious subjects, those with possible or probable anxiety were at higher risk for developing insomnia with risk ratios (RR) of 2.42 to 3.16. Elevated risk associated with anxiety remained significant even after adjusting for age, sex, social class, depression, and pain (RR = 2.13–2.43).

Morphy and colleagues[8] also examined the factors associated with persistence of insomnia over a period of 1 year. Interestingly, of all the variables included in their analysis (age, sex, social class, anxiety, depression, and pain), age was the only significant risk factor for persistence of insomnia over a period of 1 year (RR = 1.10, confidence interval [CI] = 1.03–1.18). This finding suggests that the precipitating factor for development of insomnia may be different from perpetuating factors.

Jansson-Fröjmark and Boersma[7] examined the relationship between anxiety and insomnia in a general population sample of 1498 subjects over a period of 1 year. Similar to the findings of Morphy and colleagues,[8] subjects with high anxiety in this study were significantly more likely to develop insomnia (OR = 4.27, CI = 2.63–6.94, $P<.01$) than those with low anxiety (hospital anxiety and depression scale [HADS] $\leq$7). Anxiety was also found to be an independent predictor of insomnia severity in older adults even after controlling for depression and other health-related factors.[13]

RELATIONSHIPS BETWEEN THE ONSET AND COURSE OF INSOMNIA, ANXIETY, AND DEPRESSION

- Anxiety most commonly precedes onset of insomnia.
- Insomnia most commonly occurs concurrent with or following onset of anxiety disorders.

The findings discussed previously clearly show strong associations between insomnia and anxiety and support a conceptualization of mutual risk. However, a more detailed analysis of the onset and course of insomnia in relation to anxiety provides valuable clinical insights, especially when compared with the relationship between insomnia and depression.

Ohayon and Roth[14] surveyed 14,915 subjects from the general population of several European countries regarding sleep, current psychiatric symptoms, and psychiatric history. Their findings clearly show that the insomnia-anxiety relationship differs from the insomnia-depression relationship in terms of onset and relapse in each condition. **Figs. 2** and **3** show the timing of onset of insomnia in relation to onset of first anxiety disorder and mood disorder episode, respectively.

Comparatively, insomnia is much more likely to precede the onset of mood disorders than anxiety disorders (41% vs 18%). In contrast, insomnia is much more likely to manifest concurrent with or following onset of anxiety disorders than mood disorders (83% vs 58%). The findings of Johnson and colleagues[15] largely replicated these findings with anxiety disorders occurring before the onset of insomnia in 73% of cases and insomnia occurring before the onset of depression in 69% of cases in their study.

In an attempt to determine the directionality of the effects of anxiety, insomnia, and depression on one another, Johnson and colleagues[15] performed proportional hazard analyses on the insomnia-anxiety and insomnia-depression relationship. A unique strength of this study was the inclusion of depression in the hazard models of the insomnia-anxiety relationship and vice versa, which allowed for estimation of the independent association of insomnia with each psychiatric disorder. A separate analysis was completed for (1) insomnia occurring before anxiety disorders (insomnia → anxiety disorder), (2) anxiety disorders occurring before insomnia (anxiety disorder → insomnia), and (3) insomnia occurring before major depression (insomnia → depression). **Fig. 4** provides a visual representation of these analyses.

In the insomnia → anxiety disorder analysis, the hazard ratio (HR) of prior insomnia was nonsignificant (HR = 1.6, CI = 0.7–3.5), whereas prior depression (HR = 7.0, CI = 3.0–16) and female gender (HR = 1.8, CI = 1.3–2.4) were the strongest predictors of current anxiety disorder (see **Fig. 4**). Conversely, in the anxiety disorder → insomnia analysis, only prior anxiety disorder was predictive of current insomnia (HR = 3.5, CI = 2.3–5.5; see **Fig. 4**). In the insomnia → depression analysis, prior insomnia (CI = 3.8. CI = 1.6–8.6) and prior

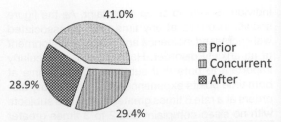

Fig. 3. Onset of insomnia in relation to onset of first mood disorder episode. (*Data from* Ohayon MM, Roth T. Place of chronic insomnia in the course of depressive and anxiety disorders. J Psychiatr Res 2003;37:9–15.)

anxiety (HR = 2.8, CI = 1.3–5.7) were each significant predictors of current depression (see **Fig. 4**).

Based on their findings and those of the longitudinal epidemiologic studies discussed previously, Ohayon and Roth[14] proposed that, in many cases, anxiety represents an etiologic factor for depression with the combination of insomnia and anxiety leading to depression. Other studies have also identified anxiety as an independent risk factor for depression.[16] The findings of Johnson and colleagues[15] as depicted in **Fig. 4** appear to support this conclusion.

THERAPEUTIC OPTIONS AND CLINICAL OUTCOMES

- Pharmacotherapy and cognitive-behavior therapy are each effective for the treatment of anxiety and insomnia.
- Monotherapy for anxiety has a moderate effect on insomnia symptoms. However, residual insomnia symptoms are common despite remission of anxiety symptoms.

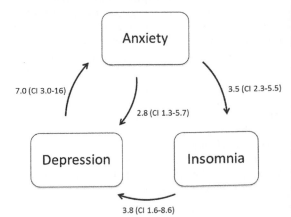

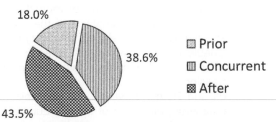

Fig. 2. Onset of insomnia in relation to onset of first anxiety disorder. (*Data from* Ohayon MM, Roth T. Place of chronic insomnia in the course of depressive and anxiety disorders. J Psychiatr Res 2003;37:9–15.)

Fig. 4. Direction and magnitude of risk of insomnia, anxiety, and depression associated with prior onset of each condition respectively. (*Data from* Johnson EO, Roth T, Breslau N. The association of insomnia with anxiety disorders and depression: exploration of the direction of risk. J Psychiatr Res 2006;40:700–8.)

- Monotherapy for insomnia has a moderate effect on anxiety symptoms.
- Combination therapy for anxiety and insomnia leads to improved sleep and augmented anxiety outcomes.

Crossover Effects of Monotherapies

Treatment outcome studies provide an empirical basis for judgments regarding the relationship between anxiety and insomnia. Belleville and colleagues[17,18] have recently published findings of 2 meta-analyses of the effect of cognitive behavioral therapy (CBT) for anxiety disorders on insomnia and vice versa. Of 1205 studies investigating CBT for anxiety disorders, only 25 reported data on sleep variables. Based on their analysis of these 25 studies, CBT for anxiety disorders has a moderate effect on insomnia (combined effect size [ES] = 0.527, CI = 0.306–0.748). Conversely, based on their analysis of 216 cognitive-behavioral therapy for insomnia (CBT-I) trials, they found that CBT-I has a moderate effect on anxiety (combined ES = 0.406, CI = 0.318–0.493). With these findings in mind, it is reasonable to expect that monotherapy for insomnia or anxiety may result in resolution of both conditions in some cases. However, the moderate ESs in each study suggest that persistence of clinically significant residual symptoms is just as likely.

Residual Insomnia Symptoms Following Monotherapy for Anxiety

Numerous treatment studies have found insomnia to be a common residual symptom following effective treatment of many anxiety disorders. Forty-eight percent (13 of 27) of posttraumatic stress disorders (PTSD) patients continued to report insomnia despite no longer meeting PTSD criteria following CBT.[19] Thirty percent (8 of 27) of subjects in this study continued to meet criteria for severe insomnia, which was defined as 90 minutes or more of lost sleep "several days per week." Cervena and colleagues[20] examined the changes in insomnia symptoms as measured by sleep logs, questionnaires, and polysomnography (PSG) in panic disorder patients following 8 weeks of combined pharmacotherapy and CBT. Despite statistically significant improvements in anxiety and depression symptoms and clinical global impression (CGI) scores, no statistically significant changes were documented for sleep onset latency (SOL), total sleep time, sleep quality, or feeling "refreshed" in the mornings. Although statistically significant changes were documented in PSG recorded sleep stages 1 and 4 sleep, the clinical relevance of these changes for insomnia complaints is questionable given the lack of improvements in subjective ratings.

Insomnia Improves with Administration of Targeted Treatment

Multiple well-designed clinical trials of CBT-I have established that insomnia symptoms improve in response to targeted intervention regardless of medical or psychiatric comorbidity.[21] In a study comparing response to CBT-I for insomnia in patients with primary insomnia versus insomnia associated with mixed psychiatric disorders, patients with comorbid insomnia responded to CBT-I as well as patients with primary insomnia.[22] There were no statistically significant differences in ESs for the primary insomnia versus comorbid insomnia groups on sleep diary measures of SOL or sleep efficiency; wake after sleep onset as measured by actigraphy; or insomnia symptoms, subjective sleep quality, or disruptive sleep-related beliefs as measured by outcome questionnaires.

Combination Therapies Improve Insomnia and Augment Anxiety Outcomes

Recent clinical trials of combination therapies for chronic insomnia and anxiety disorders have found improved insomnia and augmented anxiolytic outcomes with combination versus monotherapies. Pollack and colleagues[23] completed a 10-week, double-blind, placebo-controlled trial of eszopiclone coadministered with escitalopram in patients with comorbid chronic insomnia and generalized anxiety disorder. Compared with placebo, the eszopiclone group experienced larger improvements in insomnia, depression, and anxiety symptoms as measured by several well-validated patient and clinician rating scales (eg, Insomnia Severity Index, HADS, Hamilton Anxiety and Depression Scales [HAM-A, HAM-D], and multiple CGI scales). The advantage for the eszopiclone group on sleep measures was lost following discontinuation of eszopiclone. However, the eszopiclone group continued to experience greater improvements in anxiety symptoms compared with the placebo group even after eszopiclone was discontinued.

A similar study examining escitalopram combined with zolpidem extended-release demonstrated similar results for sleep variables during active treatment and following discontinuation of zolpidem.[24] However, in this study, cotherapy with zolpidem demonstrated no advantage over placebo on any anxiety variable. Gross and colleagues[25] performed an open-label study of ramelteon as an adjunct to selective serotonin reuptake inhibitor (SSRI)/serotonin-norepinephrine reuptake inhibitor (SNRI) treatment in patients with generalized anxiety disorder (GAD) who were partially responsive to SSRI/SNRI monotherapy. Within-group comparisons of pretreatment and post-treatment symptoms documented statistically significant improvements in sleep and anxiety as measured by sleep diaries, HAM-A, and multiple CGI scales.

From these 3 studies, it can be tentatively concluded that hypnotic cotherapy does improve sleep during active use of the hypnotic. However, sleep-related treatment gains are not sustained following discontinuation of the hypnotic. In addition, although cotherapy with eszopiclone and ramelteon was associated with augmentation of the anxiolytic effects of primary antidepressant pharmacotherapy, this anxiolytic augmentation was not seen with use of zolpidem as cotherapy.

Putative Mechanisms of Anxiolytic Augmentation with Insomnia Pharmacotherapy

It has been suggested that the advantage for eszopiclone over zolpidem in terms of anxiolytic effect may be the result of each drug's unique profile of γ-aminobutyric acid A (GABA$_A$) receptor subtype selectivity.[26] However, given the lack of GABA action by ramelteon, either the anxiolytic effects must not be related to GABA action or the GABA action may represent one of multiple pathways to anxiolytic effects associated with treatment of comorbid insomnia. In fact, Gross and colleagues[25] attribute the anxiolytic effect of adjunctive use of ramelteon directly to the marked increase in total sleep time documented in their study.

COMPLICATIONS AND CONCERNS
The Issue of Diagnostic Reliability and Validity

The reliability and validity of diagnostic categories of psychiatric disorders established in current nosologies are a matter of vigorous and ongoing debate; this is also true for anxiety and insomnia disorder diagnoses specifically. In their recent review of the epidemiology of anxiety disorders, Kessler and colleagues[2] suggest that current classification systems for anxiety disorders are not supported by epidemiologic and factor analytical studies. Relatively sophisticated studies of insomnia diagnoses from 2 independent groups using different methodologies have produced findings that significantly bring into question the reliability, validity, and clinical utility of the insomnia diagnoses specified in current nosologies.[27,28] In consideration of this, investigations of insomnia and anxiety as manifested at both the symptom

and the diagnostic level have been included in the current review.

The Issue of Age-of-Onset and Age-of-Assessment

Emerging opinion supports the potentially critical role of both the age-of-onset and the age-of-assessment in the diagnosis and treatment of comorbid insomnia, anxiety, and depression. Age-of-onset of anxiety disorders is predominantly in childhood or adolescence, making them the temporally primary disorders in most cases of psychiatric comorbidity.[2] In addition, initial assessment and treatment of anxiety disorders often do not occur for more than a decade following initial onset.[2] Based on their review of existing research and their own original findings, Gregory and colleagues[29] suggest that age may be a prominent factor in the association between anxiety, depression, and insomnia. Uhde and colleagues[10] take the issue of age-of-onset and age-of-assessment one step further, stating that resolution of insomnia through treatment of comorbid anxiety can be expected, "…only if treatment were initiated at the earliest phase of illness."

SUMMARY

Concurrent clinical presentation of insomnia and anxiety is frequent in clinical practice. The onset and course of anxiety and insomnia are intimately related, and traditional conceptualizations of insomnia as secondary to anxiety are no longer clinically viable. An evolving body of evidence suggests a relationship between these 2 conditions that is complex and reciprocal and that evolves over time. In terms of diagnosis and management, unless initial assessment and intervention are initiated in the earliest stages of illness, emerging opinion supports recognition of co-occurring anxiety and insomnia as independent comorbid conditions, with each condition likely requiring targeted therapeutic attention to achieve optimal therapeutic outcomes.

REFERENCES

1. Breslau N, Roth T, Rosenthal L, et al. Sleep disturbance and psychiatric disorders: a longitudinal epidemiological study of young adults. Biol Psychiatry 1996;39:411–8.
2. Kessler RC, Ruscio AM, Shear K, et al. Epidemiology of anxiety disorders. Curr Top Behav Neurosci 2010;2:21–35.
3. Ford DE, Kamerow DB. Epidemiologic study of sleep disturbances and psychiatric disorders. An opportunity for prevention? JAMA 1989;262:1479–84.

4. Ohayon MM. Observation of the natural evolution of insomnia in the American general population cohort. Sleep Med Clin 2009;4:87–92.

5. Pollack M, Seal B, Joish VN, et al. Insomnia-related comorbidities and economic costs among a commercially insured population in the United States. Curr Med Res Opin 2009;25:1901–11.

6. Ramsawh HJ, Stein MB, Belik SL, et al. Relationship of anxiety disorders, sleep quality, and functional impairment in a community sample. J Psychiatr Res 2009;43:926–33.

7. Jansson-Fröjmark M, Boersma K. Bidirectionality between pain and insomnia symptoms: a prospective study. Br J Health Psychol 2012;17:420–31.

8. Morphy H, Dunn KM, Lewis M, et al. Epidemiology of insomnia: a longitudinal study in a UK population. Sleep 2007;30:274–80.

9. Marcks BA, Weisberg RB, Edelen MO, et al. The relationship between sleep disturbance and the course of anxiety disorders in primary care patients. Psychiatry Res 2010;178:487–92.

10. Uhde TW, Cortese BM, Vedeniapin A. Anxiety and sleep problems: emerging concepts and theoretical treatment implications. Curr Psychiatry Rep 2009; 11:269–76.

11. National Institutes of Health. National Institutes of Health State of the Science Conference statement on manifestations and management of chronic insomnia in adults, June 13–15, 2005. Sleep 2005; 28:1049–57.

12. Taylor DJ, Lichstein KL, Durrence HH, et al. Epidemiology of insomnia, depression, and anxiety. Sleep 2005;28:1457–64.

13. Botts E, Orr W, Glidewell R. Influence of anxiety on insomnia in older adults when controlling for depression. Sleep 2009;32:A357.

14. Ohayon MM, Roth T. Place of chronic insomnia in the course of depressive and anxiety disorders. J Psychiatr Res 2003;37:9–15.

15. Johnson EO, Roth T, Breslau N. The association of insomnia with anxiety disorders and depression: exploration of the direction of risk. J Psychiatr Res 2006;40:700–8.

16. Goodwin RD. Anxiety disorders and the onset of depression among adults in the community. Psychol Med 2002;32:1121–4.

17. Belleville G, Cousineau H, Levrier K, et al. The impact of cognitive-behavior therapy for anxiety disorders on concomitant sleep disturbances: a meta-analysis. J Anxiety Disord 2010;24:379–86.

18. Belleville G, Cousineau H, Levrier K, et al. Meta-analytic review of the impact of cognitive-behavior therapy for insomnia on concomitant anxiety. Clin Psychol Rev 2011;31:638–52.

19. Zayfert C, DeViva JC. Residual insomnia following cognitive behavioral therapy for PTSD. J Trauma Stress 2004;17:69–73.

20. Cervena K, Matousek M, Prasko J, et al. Sleep disturbances in patients treated for panic disorder. Sleep Med 2005;6:149–53.

21. Smith MT, Huang MI, Manber R. Cognitive behavior therapy for chronic insomnia occurring within the context of medical and psychiatric disorders. Clin Psychol Rev 2005;25:559–92.

22. Edinger JD, Olsen MK, Stechuchak KM, et al. Cognitive behavioral therapy for patients with primary insomnia or insomnia associated predominantly with mixed psychiatric disorders: a randomized clinical trial. Sleep 2009;32:499–510.

23. Pollack M, Kinrys G, Krystal A, et al. Eszopiclone co-administered with escitalopram in patients with insomnia and comorbid generalized anxiety disorder. Arch Gen Psychiatry 2008;65:551–62.

24. Fava M, Asnis GM, Shrivastava R, et al. Zolpidem extended-release improves sleep and next-day symptoms in comorbid insomnia and generalized anxiety disorder. J Clin Psychopharmacol 2009;29:222–30.

25. Gross PK, Nourse R, Wasser TE. Ramelteon for insomnia symptoms in a community sample of adults with generalized anxiety disorder: an open label study. J Clin Sleep Med 2009;5:28–33.

26. Fava M, Schaefer K, Huang H, et al. A post hoc analysis of the effect of nightly administration of eszopiclone and a selective serotonin reuptake inhibitor in patients with insomnia and anxious depression. J Clin Psychiatry 2011;72:473–9.

27. Edinger JD, Wyatt JK, Stepanski EJ, et al. Testing the reliability and validity of DSM-IV-TR and ICSD-2 insomnia diagnoses. Results of a multitrait-multimethod analysis. Arch Gen Psychiatry 2011;68: 992–1002.

28. Ohayon MM, Reynolds CF. Epidemiological and clinical relevance of insomnia diagnosis algorithms according to the DSM-IV and the International Classification of Sleep Disorders (ICSD). Sleep Med 2009;10:952–60.

29. Gregory AM, Rijsdijk FV, Dahl RE, et al. Associations between sleep problems, anxiety, and depression in twins at 8 years of age. Pediatrics 2006;118: 1124–32.

Interventions for Sleep Disturbance in Bipolar Disorder

Allison G. Harvey, PhD[a,*], Katherine A. Kaplan, PhD[b],
Adriane M. Soehner, PhD[c]

KEYWORDS

• Bipolar disorder • Sleep disturbances • Psychological interventions

KEY POINTS

- Sleep disturbance is associated with decreased quality of life and mood relapse in bipolar disorder.
- Sleep disturbance persists at high rates in bipolar disorder despite adequate pharmacologic treatment for mood disturbance.
- Cognitive behavioral therapy for insomnia leads to clinically significant and sustained improvement in sleep for chronic insomniacs.
- Adjunctive nonpharmacological sleep intervention, drawing upon principles from cognitive behavioral therapy for insomnia, interpersonal and social rhythm therapy, and motivational interviewing, is a viable treatment for sleep disturbance in bipolar disorder.
- Psychological interventions for sleep disturbance are advantageous in that they have few adverse effects, may be preferred by patients, are durable, and have no abuse potential.

INTERVENTIONS FOR SLEEP DISTURBANCE IN BIPOLAR DISORDER

Bipolar disorder is a common, severe, and chronic disorder. It is often life-threatening, with approximately 1 in 5 individuals completing suicide.[1] The lifetime prevalence of Bipolar I and II is 1% and 0.5%, respectively,[2] although more liberal definitions of hypomania identify many more patients with bipolar spectrum disorder. Bipolar disorder type I is defined by the presence of at least 1 manic or mixed episode. Bipolar II requires at least 1 hypomanic episode and at least 1 major depressive episode.[2] The impact that episodes of mania or depression have on the person's life is enormous. After the onset of the disorder, individuals with bipolar disorder who have been hospitalized spend approximately 20% of their life in episodes[3] and approximately 50% of their time unwell.[4] Not surprisingly, bipolar disorder is ranked as one of the top 10 leading causes of disability worldwide.

There have been important advances in pharmacologic and nonpharmacologic treatments for bipolar disorder. However, even with continued adherence, many patients remain seriously symptomatic in the interepisode period,[5] and the risk of relapse over 5 years is as high as 73%.[6] In response to these high relapse rates, research continues to try to improve pharmacotherapy and also to develop adjunctive psychosocial treatments.[7] The latter include interpersonal and social rhythm therapy (IPSRT), family therapy, psychoeducation and cognitive behavior therapy (CBT) administered individually or in groups, as well as combination approaches. Even with the

a Department of Psychology, University of California, Berkeley, Berkeley, CA 94720-1650, USA; b Department of Psychiatry, Stanford University School of Medicine, Psychiatry and Behavioral Sciences, 401 Quarry Road, Stanford, CA 94305-5722, USA; c Department of Psychiatry, University of Pittsburgh School of Medicine, Western Psychiatric Institute and Clinic, 3811 O'Hara Street, Pittsburgh, PA 15213, USA
* Corresponding author. Department of Psychology, University of California, Berkeley, 2205 Tolman Hall #1650, Berkeley, CA 94720-1650.
E-mail address: aharvey@berkeley.edu

Sleep Med Clin 10 (2015) 101–105
http://dx.doi.org/10.1016/j.jsmc.2014.11.005
1556-407X/15/$ – see front matter © 2015 Elsevier Inc. All rights reserved.

combination of pharmacologic and adjunctive interventions, the rates of relapse remain of concern, and many individuals remain highly symptomatic between episodes.[7]

WHY IS SLEEP IMPORTANT IN BIPOLAR DISORDER?
Bipolar Disorder and Sleep Disturbance Often Coexist

Reduced need for sleep is a classic symptom of mania. During episodes of depression, insomnia, or hypersomnia are common. Even in the interepisode period, sleep is disturbed; up to 70% of bipolar disorder patients report insomnia,[8] which is associated with risk for relapse and suicide attempts.[9] Hypersomnia is experienced by roughly 25% of bipolar 1 patients during the interepisode period,[10] and by 40% to 80% of these patients during episodes of depression.[11] Sleep disturbance is characteristic across the bipolar spectrum. In fact, total sleep time is shortest in bipolar disorder–not otherwise specified, relative to bipolar 1 disorder and bipolar 2 disorder, but the 3 subtypes are equally impaired in night-to-night variability.[12] Mean variability in total sleep time across a week in bipolar patients is approximately 2.78 hours (SD = 3.02),[12] almost equivalent to flying from the east to west coast of continents like North America and Australia. The human circadian rhythm cannot easily adapt to these fast shifts. Indeed, in interepisode bipolar disorder, lower and more variable sleep efficiency and variability in falling asleep time are related to worse illness course and outcome.[13] Relative to the interepisode phase, sleep disturbance escalates just before an episode, worsens during an episode,[14–16] and does not always resolve with medication. Among individuals treated with best practice mood stabilizers in Systematic Treatment Enhancement Program for Bipolar Disorder (STEP-BD),[17] 66% still experienced significant sleep disturbance.[12,18]

Sleep Disturbance Contributes to Affective Dysregulation

Multiple studies suggest that sleep disturbance contributes to affective dysregulation in bipolar disorder:

a. Sleep disturbance is a common prodrome of relapse.[16]
b. Short sleepers exhibited more symptoms of mania, depression, anxiety and irritability, lower scores on functioning and life satisfaction compared with bipolar disorder patients with longer sleep times.[12] Moreover, shorter total

sleep time was associated with increased mania and depression severity over 12 months[18]
c. In a 7-day diary study, total wake time was associated with next-day morning negative mood in bipolar disorder, while evening negative mood was associated with subsequent total wake time in both bipolar disorder and insomnia[19]
d. Experimentally-induced sleep deprivation is associated with the onset of hypomania or mania[15]
e. Sleep has a critical mood regulatory function, and sleep deprivation involves the loss of top-down inhibitory control usually exerted by medial prefrontal cortex on amygdala[20]
f. Circuits involved in emotion regulation and sleep regulation interact in bidirectional ways.[21] In sum, sleep disturbance is a pathway leading to affective instability and relapse by means of well-recognized neural circuits.

Sleep Disturbance Contributes to Interepisode Functional Impairment

Even with good adherence to medication, many patients with bipolar disorder remain seriously symptomatic in the interepisode period. Clinically significant insomnia is one of the most common residual symptoms.[8] Insomnia in itself has a significant negative psychosocial, occupational, health, and economic impact.[22] The authors' analysis of STEP-BD data indicates that sleeping less than 6.5 hours per night is associated with greater symptom severity and greater impairment relative to sleeping 6.5 to 8.5 hours.[18]

Taken together these, data highlight the complexity and multiple sleep disturbances that are characteristic of bipolar disorder (insomnia, hypersomnia, delayed sleep phase, irregular sleep–wake schedule, reduced sleep need) and the importance of an intervention to improve sleep as a pathway for improvement of mood and reducing impairment.

MANAGING SLEEP DISTURBANCE IN BIPOLAR DISORDER

Pharmacologic treatment of bipolar disorder is inseparable from the treatment of sleep disturbance. Here the focus is on describing a nonpharmacologic approach because

1. There are fewer adverse effects or interactions with other treatments for the bipolar disorder and other conditions
2. Although hypnotics are efficacious and clinically indicated in some situations (eg, acute insomnia), concerns remain about the durability,

daytime residual effects, tolerance, dependence, and rebound insomnia
3. Given the comorbidity between bipolar disorder and substance use disorders,[23] certain classes of insomnia medications—most important, the US Food and Drug Administration (FDA)-approved benzodiazepine receptor agonists—pose a risk of abuse.

As already mentioned, several psychological adjunctive interventions have been developed for patients with bipolar disorder including IPSRT, family therapy, CBT, and psychoeducation. Each of these includes at least 1 component designed to target sleep. However, specific sleep outcomes have not been reported, and these treatments have yet to draw from advances in knowledge of the effectiveness of CBT for insomnia (CBT-I). Evidence documenting the efficacy of CBT-I for patients with chronic insomnia (ie, nonbipolar insomnia patients) has been summarized in several quantitative and systematic reviews of the literature, including 3 meta analyses and 2 review/practice parameter papers commissioned by the American Academy of Sleep Medicine.[24] These sleep improvements are well sustained up to 2 years after cessation of treatment.[25] Evidence is accruing to suggest that insomnia that co-occurs with a range of psychiatric disorders can be improved with CBT-I. Hence, the treatment approach described draws on CBT-I. The unique features of sleep disturbance in bipolar disorder led to modifications of typical CBT-I procedures and the addition of elements from IPSRT[26] and motivational interviewing (MI).[27] However, it should be noted that this approach is being evaluated for bipolar disorder, and there has been a need to adapt some components for use with bipolar patients.

Functional Analysis/Case Formulation and Goal Setting

The frequency, intensity, and duration of insomnia and its antecedents are discussed. Sleep-related behaviors and consequences are assessed: before bed (eg, bedtime routine), during the night (eg, cell phone left on), on waking (eg, sleepiness, lethargy) and during the day (eg, caffeine use). The relationship between sleep-specific thoughts, emotions, and behaviors is charted across the night and day. Specific goals are identified (eg, increase total sleep time or earlier lights out time).

Motivational Interviewing

A straightforward review of perceived pros and cons of the change is conducted, recognizing that many sleep-incompatible/interfering behaviors are rewarding. For example, patients often struggle with waking up at around the same time weekdays and weekends. Allowing the patient to generate advantages and disadvantages with therapist guidance facilitates behavior change. MI is revisited in future sessions as additional strategies are introduced.

Sleep and Circadian Education

Education relevant to the circadian system includes definitions, explanation of environmental influences (particularly light), the importance of circadian and social rhythms (following IPSRT), and the tendency to drift toward a delayed sleep phase. Sleep inertia, or the subjective feeling of grogginess after awakening, is defined and normalized. Sleep disturbance is identified as a common prodrome of relapse. A link is drawn between sleep disturbance and daytime mood dysfunction, including the mood regulatory function of sleep. Finally, the authors highlight the different behavioral strategies needed for treatment of the current sleep problem and for sleep problems in the future (eg, hypersomnia, reduced sleep need, delayed phase). In later sessions, the authors return to this topic and adapt each sleep principle so patients have a well-developed decision tree and menu of options for managing the range of sleep problems they may experience.

Behavioral Components

Stimulus control
One of the most effective treatment components of CBT-I,[24] stimulus control focuses on regularizing the sleep–wake cycle and strengthening associations between the bed and sleep.[28] For certain patients, the authors adapt the instruction to get out of bed if it risks hem engaging in rewarding and arousing activities that prevent sleep.

Restricting time in bed
Restricting time in bed[29] is derived from the observation that excessive time in bed perpetuates insomnia. The authors limit time in bed to the actual time slept, and gradually increase it back to an optimal sleep time. In order to avoid changes in mood related to short-term sleep deprivation, minimum time in bed is never lower than 6.5 hours, and the authors carefully monitor mood for changes in manic/hypomanic symptoms. The goal is to maximize sleep efficiency to greater than 85% to 90%. More consolidated sleep is experienced as more satisfying.

Regularizing sleep and wake times

IPSRT is utilized to regularize sleep and wake times across the week. Building motivation for the patient to wake at the same time (including on weekends[30]) is a key focus. This promotes consistent sleepiness in the evening, particularly when naps are avoided, and enables patients with a tendency toward eveningness to progressively move their bedtime forward by 20–30 minutes per week (small enough that the circadian system can adapt).

Wind-down

Patients need assistance to devise a wind-down of 30 to 60 minutes, in which relaxing, sleep-enhancing activities are introduced, in dim light conditions. This helps the circadian phase advance in patients who are evening-types, and maintains entrainment.[31] A central issue is the use of interactive electronic media (Internet, cell phones, MP3 players). MI and behavioral experiments are used to facilitate voluntarily choosing an electronic curfew, recognizing that many patients are socially isolated and rely on prebedtime Internet-based social interaction. Many patients prefer to set an alarm on a cell phone to remind themselves of this curfew.

Wake-up

This individualized intervention draws on principles from IPSRT and includes: not hitting snooze, opening the curtains to let sunlight in, spending the first 30 to 60 minutes after waking outside or in a room with bright lights, encouraging morning activity and social contact to counteract sleep inertia, and making the bed so the incentive to get back in is reduced.

Cognitive Components

Challenging unhelpful beliefs

Challenging unhelpful beliefs about sleep is important.[32] Unhelpful beliefs about sleep are common in bipolar disorder[8] and include: 'there is no point going to bed earlier, because I won't be able to fall asleep,' 'the TV helps me fall asleep,' and 'medication is the only thing that contributes to my feeling drowsy.' Guided discovery and individualized experiments test the validity and utility of the beliefs.[33]

Anxiety

Patients with bipolar disorder are anxious about their sleep, in part because they know that sleep loss can herald a relapse.[8] As anxiety is antithetical to sleep onset, the authors use individualized strategies to reduce bedtime worry, rumination, and vigilance including cognitive therapy, diary writing, or scheduling a worry period.

Monitoring

Bipolar patients with disturbed sleep often monitor for signs of fatigue upon waking or throughout the day. Helping the patient understand that feeling groggy upon waking is normal (sleep inertia), and introducing behavioral experiments and attention strategies for monitoring in the daytime, can reduce anxiety and preoccupation with sleep.

Daytime Coping

Patients with bipolar disorder typically believe the only way they can feel less tired in the daytime is to sleep more. Hence, a behavioral experiment is devised to allow the patient to experience the energy-generating effects of activity.[33] This is also an opportunity to develop a list of energy-generating and energy-sapping activities that can be used to manage daytime tiredness, the postlunch circadian dip in alertness, and build resilience to inevitable bouts of occasional sleep deprivation.

Relapse Prevention

The goal is to consolidate skills and prepare for setbacks. Patients and therapists together discuss potential obstacles to maintaining gains and problem solve around areas of future sleep disturbance. An individualized summary of learning and achievements guides relapse prevention work. Areas needing further intervention are addressed by setting specific goals and creating plans for achieving each goal.

REFERENCES

1. Isometsä ET. Course, outcome, and suicide risk in bipolar disorder: a review. Psychiatr Fennica 1993; 24:113–24.
2. American Psychiatric Association. Task force on DSM-IV. Diagnostic and statistical manual of mental disorders: DSM-IV-TR. 4th edition. Washington, DC: American Psychiatric Association; 2000.
3. Angst J, Sellaro R. Historical perspectives and natural history of bipolar disorder. Biol Psychiatry 2000; 48:445–57.
4. Joffe RT, MacQueen GM, Marriott M, et al. A prospective, longitudinal study of percentage of time spent ill in patients with bipolar I or bipolar II disorders. Bipolar Disord 2004;6:62–6.
5. MacQueen GM, Marriott M, Begin H, et al. Subsyndromal symptoms assessed in longitudinal, prospective follow-up of a cohort of patients with bipolar disorder. Bipolar Disord 2003;5:349–55.
6. Gitlin MJ, Swendsen J, Heller TL, et al. Relapse and impairment in bipolar disorder. Am J Psychiatry 1995;152:1635–40.

7. Craighead WE, Miklowitz DJ, Frank E, et al. Psychosocial treatments for bipolar disorder. In: Nathan PE, Gorman JM, editors. A guide to treatments that work. 2nd edition. London: Oxford University Press; 2002. p. 263–75.

8. Harvey AG, Schmidt DA, Scarna A, et al. Sleep-related functioning in euthymic patients with bipolar disorder, patients with insomnia, and subjects without sleep problems. Am J Psychiatry 2005;162:50–7.

9. Sylvia LG, Dupuy JM, Ostacher MJ, et al. Sleep disturbance in euthymic bipolar patients. J Psychopharmacol 2012;26:1108–12.

10. Kaplan KA, Gruber J, Eidelman P, et al. Hypersomnia in inter-episode bipolar disorder: does it have prognostic significance? J Affect Disord 2011; 132(3):438–44.

11. Kaplan KA, Harvey AG. Hypersomnia across mood disorders: a review and synthesis. Sleep Med Rev 2009;13(4):275–85.

12. Gruber J, Harvey AG, Wang PW, et al. Sleep functioning in relation to mood, function, and quality of life at entry to the Systematic Treatment Enhancement Program for Bipolar Disorder (STEP-BD). J Affect Disord 2009;114:41–9.

13. Eidelman P, Talbot LS, Gruber J, et al. Sleep, illness course, and concurrent symptoms in inter-episode bipolar disorder. J Behav Ther Exp Psychiatry 2010;41:145–9.

14. American Psychiatric Association. Diagnostic and statistical manual of mental disorders. 4th edition, text revision. Washington, DC: American Psychiatric Association; 2000.

15. Wehr TA, Sack DA, Rosenthal NE. Sleep reduction as a final common pathway in the genesis of mania. Am J Psychiatry 1987;144:201–4.

16. Jackson A, Cavanagh J, Scott J. A systematic review of manic and depressive prodromes. J Affect Disord 2003;74:209–17.

17. Sachs GS, Thase ME, Otto MW, et al. Rationale, design, and methods of the systematic treatment enhancement program for bipolar disorder (STEP-BD). Biol Psychiatry 2003;53:1028–42.

18. Gruber J, Miklowitz DJ, Harvey AG, et al. Sleep matters: sleep functioning and course of illness in bipolar disorder. J Affect Disord 2011;134:416–20.

19. Talbot L, Stone S, Gruber J, et al. A test of the bidirectional association between sleep and mood in bipolar disorder and insomnia. J Abnorm Psychol 2012;121(1):39–50.

20. Yoo S, Gujar N, Hu P, et al. The human emotional brain without sleep: a prefrontal-amygdala disconnect? Curr Biol 2007;17:R877–8.

21. Saper CB, Cano G, Scammell TE. Homeostatic, circadian, and emotional regulation of sleep. J Comp Neurol 2005;493:92–8.

22. Ancoli-Israel S, Roth T. Characteristics of insomnia in the United States: results of the 1991 National Sleep Foundation Survey. I. Sleep 1999;22(Suppl 2):S347–53.

23. Levin FR, Hennessy G. Bipolar disorder and substance abuse. Biol Psychiatry 2004;56:738–48.

24. Morin CM, Bootzin RR, Buysse DJ, et al. Psychological and behavioral treatment of insomnia: an update of recent evidence (1998–2004). Sleep 2006;29: 1396–406.

25. Morin CM, Colecchi C, Stone J, et al. Behavioral and pharmacological therapies for late-life insomnia. J Am Med Assoc 1999;281:991–9.

26. Frank E, Swartz HA, Kupfer DJ. Interpersonal and social rhythm therapy: managing the chaos of bipolar disorder. Biol Psychiatry 2000;48:593–604.

27. Miller WR, Rollnick S. Motivational interviewing: preparing people for change. New York: Guilford Press; 2002.

28. Bootzin RR. Stimulus control treatment for insomnia. Proceedings American Psychological Association 1972;7:395–6.

29. Spielman AJ, Saskin P, Thorpy MJ. Treatment of chronic insomnia by restriction of time in bed. Sleep 1987;10:45–56.

30. Crowley SJ, Carskadon MA. Modifications to weekend recovery sleep delay circadian phase in older adolescents. Chronobiol Int 2010;27:1469–92.

31. Wyatt JK, Stepanski EJ, Kirkby J. Circadian phase in delayed sleep phase syndrome: predictors and temporal stability across multiple assessments. Sleep 2006;29:1075–80.

32. Edinger JD, Wohlgemuth WK, Radtke RA, et al. Does cognitive–behavioral insomnia therapy alter dysfunctional beliefs about sleep? Sleep 2001;24: 591–9.

33. Ree M, Harvey AG. Insomnia. In: Bennett-Levy J, Butler G, Fennell M, et al, editors. Oxford guide to behavioural experiments in cognitive therapy. Oxford (England): Oxford University Press; 2004. p. 287–305.

Printed and bound by CPI Group (UK) Ltd, Croydon, CR0 4YY

03/10/2024

01040366-0003